T0140779

Signal processing concepts for the assessment of coronary plaques with intravascular ultrasound

Christian Perrey

Bibliografische Information Der Deutschen Bibliothek

Die Deutsche Bibliothek verzeichnet diese Publikation in der Deutschen Nationalbibliografie; detaillierte bibliografische Daten sind im Internet über http://dnb.ddb.de abrufbar.

ISBN 3-8325-1233-0

Logos Verlag Berlin
Comeniushof, Gubener Str. 47,
10243 Berlin
Tel.: +49 030 42 85 10 90
Fax: +49 030 42 85 10 92
INTERNET: http://www.logos-verlag.de

Signal processing concepts for the assessment of coronary plaques with intravascular ultrasound

DISSERTATION

zur Erlangung des Grades eines
Doktor-Ingenieurs
der Fakultät für Elektrotechnik
und Informationstechnik
der Ruhr-Universität Bochum

von
Christian Perrey
Recklinghausen

Bochum 2005

Tag der mündlichen Prüfung:	24. Juni 2005
Berichter:	Prof. Dr.-Ing. Helmut Ermert
	Prof. Dr.-Ing. Werner von Seelen

Contents

Symbols and Acronyms

Greek symbols

α	angle between mechanical strain and ultrasound beam
α_w	weight for calculation of $E_{internal}$
β_w	weight for calculation of $E_{internal}$
γ_w	weight for calculation of E_{image}
δ	angle of catheter tilt
δ_{ce}	angle of catheter eccentricity
δ_{ax}	axial resolution
δ_{lat}	lateral resolution
δ_w	weight for calculation of E_{image}
ε	mechanical strain
ε_r, ε_Θ, ε_z	radial, circumferential and longitudinal mechanical strain
ζ	elevation angle of the imaging geometry
Θ	azimuth angle of the vessel geometry
λ	wavelength
μ	mean value
ν	Poisson's ratio
$\mathbf{v}(s)$	contour vector
$\mathbf{\upsilon}_i$	vector to a discrete point on a contour
$\rho(r,\varphi)$	normalized correlation coefficient
σ_r, σ_Θ, σ_z	radial, circumferential and longitudinal mechanical stress
σ	standard deviation
σ^2_τ	variance of time delay estimation
σ^2_ε	strain variance
τ	time shift between two signals
φ	azimuth angle of the imaging geometry
φ_j	discrete azimuth angle (for synthetic aperture focusing)
$\varphi(t)$	signal phase
ω	angular frequency
ω_0	angular center frequency

Latin symbols

A_{ROC}	Area under the ROC curve
B	bandwith
$b_{n,m}$	image brightness amplitude
c	speed of sound
C_{aa}, C_{dd}	power spectra of blood pressure signals

C_{ad}	cross spectrum of blood pressure signals
dB	decibel
E	elastic modulus
$E(\upsilon)$	snake energy functional
$E_{internal}$	internal energy of a contour (snake)
E_{image}	Energy due to image forces
E_{con}	Energy due to external constraint forces
f	frequency
f_0	center frequency
f_s	sampling frequency
Δf_{-6dB}	-6 dB bandwidth
$E(\upsilon)$	snake energy functional
$I(r,\varphi)$	image intensity
N_A	number of elements in a transducer array sub-aperture
N_d	distance between signal window segments
N_e	number of elements in a transducer array
N_s	window size of least squares differentiator filter
N_w	signal window size
O	computational complexity
p	pressure
p_a	blood pressure proximal of a stenosis
$\bar{p}_a$	mean blood pressure proximal of a stenosis
p_d	blood pressure distal of a stenosis
$\bar{p}_d$	mean blood pressure distal of a stenosis
Δp	blood pressure difference
$\Delta \bar{p}$	mean blood pressure difference
$P_{d,n}(i,j)$	co-occurence matrix
r	radial distance
$R_{ad}(f)$	coherence function
R_{mean}	mean value of the coherence function
r_i	discrete radial distance (for synthetic aperture focusing)
r_{norm}	normalized cross correlation function at zero lag
R_0	radius of the ultrasound catheter
$r_{x1x2}(t)$	cross correlation function
s	contour arc length
T_{PRF}	pulse repetition time
T_s	sampling time
t	time
Δt_{-6dB}	-6 dB temporal width
$u(r)$	radial displacement

V	blood flow velocity
$\bar{V}$	mean blood flow velocity
W_m, W_n	Apodization window functions for beam forming
$w(z)$	longitudinal displacement
x, y, z	cartesian coordinates
$x(t)$	ultrasound echo signal
$x_+(t)$	analytic signal
$x(k)$	digitized ultrasound signal
$x_b(k)$	digitized ultrasound baseband signal
z_F	focal length

Acronyms

Acronym	Meaning
A/D	analog to digital conversion
A-line	radio frequency echo signal
A-mode	amplitude mode
B-mode	brightness mode (gray scale)
CFVR	coronary flow velocity reserve
CLRB	Cramer Rao lower bound
CON	contrast, second order texture parameter
CT	computed tomography
CW	continuous wave (doppler)
DIM	dimension, second order texture parameter
ECG	electrocardiogram
FFR	fractional flow reserve
FFT	fast fourier transform
FIR	finite impulse response
FWHM	full width half maximum
IPV	instantaneous peak flow velocity
IVUS	intravascular ultrasound
KAP	kappa, second order texture parameter
LAD	left anterior descending artery
MIN	minimum, first order texture parameter
MRI	magnetic resonance imaging
NURD	non-uniform rotational distortion
OCT	optical coherence tomography
PC	personal computer
PTCA	percutaneous transluminal coronary angioplasty
PVA	polyvinyl alcohol cryogel
PW	pulsed wave (doppler)
QCA	quantitative coronary angiography

rf	radio frequency
ROC	receiver operating characteristic
ROI	region of interest
SAD	sum of absolute difference
SAFT	synthetic aperture focusing techniques
SKEW	skewness, first order texture parameter
SNR	signal to noise ratio
SNR_e	elastographic signal to noise ratio
TGC	time gain control
VCA	voltage controlled amplifier

1 Introduction

Heart diseases are the leading cause of death in industrialized countries. In the year 2002 for instance they accounted for over 25% of all deaths in Germany [182]. The heart consists of a muscle that pumps blood through the circulatory system, arteries that supply blood to this muscle, and valves to control directional blood flow. If the function of the heart is disturbed, the cells of the body are not supplied properly with oxygen and nutrients. The consequences can be the failure of organs, leading to life threatening complications. Among the various types of heart diseases coronary artery diseases are the most common ones. They account for nearly two million deaths in Europe each year [158]. Atherosclerotic plaques are formed in the inner wall of the artery and narrow or occlude the vessel lumen. The resulting lack of blood supply may lead to a heart attack. Several imaging modalities are currently used for diagnosis of coronary diseases, the more important ones are X-ray angiography, ultrasound, computed tomography (CT), and magnetic resonance imaging (MRI). Imaging modalities are complemented by functional analysis such as coronary thermography or intravascular pressure and flow measurements.

An important invasive diagnostic tool for the assessment of coronary artery diseases is intravascular ultrasound (IVUS). It is currently regarded as the gold standard for the morphological analysis of coronary arteries. IVUS provides detailed images of normal and abnormal coronary vessel wall morphology and can be used for measuring the lumen area and plaque burden. Contrary to angiography, which only yields a planar projection view, IVUS allows a cross-sectional view of the vessel wall. Two different types of IVUS transducers are currently in clinical use: Rotating single element transducers and circular arrays. The former yield a better resolution due to higher ultrasound frequencies, but may exhibit artifacts caused by non-uniform rotational distortion (NURD). The latter do not show these artifacts, but the development of miniature arrays that yield a sufficient signal to noise ratio is challenging.

A life threatening sudden occlusion of coronary arteries is usually caused by vulnerable plaques that often cannot be identified by morphological analysis using the aforementioned imaging modalities. The composition of an atherosclerotic lesion rather than size and volume or degree of stenosis determines the risk of acute clinical events. Thus, evaluating the composition of the vessel wall and its histologic characteristics may be a key in lesion specific treatment. In this context, intravascular ultrasound (IVUS) is an important potential application for the identification of vulnerable plaques. Several methods have been developed for the characterization of vessel tissue composition with IVUS. Analysis of ultrasound gray scale images has been used to characterize carotid artery walls or coronary plaques. More advanced methods include the analysis of radio frequency (rf) data for tissue characterization or strain imaging with IVUS.

Ultrasound strain imaging is an important method for the characterization of biological tissue. In this approach the mechanical properties of tissue are evaluated. The tissue is compressed by an external force and the resulting strain is estimated from rf-echo signals acquired before and after compression using correlation techniques. The results are presented as gray scale or color coded strain images. In recent years, this method became of interest for plaque discrimination. Here, the stiffness of the tissue is evaluated to characterize vulnerable plaques, also often referred to as 'soft plaques'. Initial clinical results showed that vulnerable plaques can be identified with this method as regions exhibiting an increased strain.

In IVUS strain imaging studies conducted so far, the echo signals were stored to disk and the strain calculation was performed offline. Since IVUS is an invasive tool, the strain information should be provided during the exam to allow direct treatment. This approach requires time efficient algorithms for strain calculation. Single element transducers are the method of choice for this task, because the rf-data can be accessed easily and the high frequencies bear advantages. However, few strain imaging studies were performed yet with single element transducers. NURD is expected to degrade the correlation of consecutive images, but this effect has not been quantified yet.

The aim of this work is the development of new IVUS approaches for the assessment of coronary plaques. The major part is dedicated to the characterization of plaques by intravascular ultrasound strain imaging. Algorithms for time efficient strain estimation and vessel wall segmentation were developed and verified experimentally. As a complement, an alternative concept for the functional assessment of coronary artery stenoses was developed based on simultaneous measurements of intracoronary pressure and blood flow velocity using Doppler ultrasound.

Thesis outline

In the remainder of this chapter a more detailed medical background of coronary artery diseases is given. Furthermore, an overview of imaging methods and functional approaches for the assessment of coronary lesions is presented. Advantages and disadvantages are discussed, and the ability of these methods for plaque discrimination is reviewed. Chapter two gives an overview of IVUS imaging and transducer technology. In chapter three, strain imaging principles and applications are presented. In addition, the strain imaging algorithms used in this work are described in detail. Chapter four deals with strain imaging using array transducers. A method for the correction of geometric artifacts is presented and verified with ultrasound simulations. Furthermore, results from phantom experiments are given. Chapter five describes studies performed with rotating single element IVUS transducers. The influence of artifacts due to non-uniform rotation is evaluated in a phantom study and concepts for correction are presented. The developed strain imaging algorithms are verified with phantom experiments. The chapter concludes with strain imaging results from in vitro studies and clinical in vivo trials. Chapter six deals with the automated segmentation of coronary vessel walls, which is an important preprocessing step for IVUS strain imaging. Two alternative concepts are presented and verified with in vivo studies. Finally, chapter seven concludes this work with a study comprising intracoronary pressure and flow velocity measurements, aiming at the functional assessment of stenosis severity. From the analysis of pressure and flow measurements a parameter indicating the hemodynamic stenosis resistance is derived.

1.1 Medical Background

1.1.1 Coronary artery disease

Coronary arteries supply the heart muscle (myocardium) with blood. Similar to all arteries they consist of three concentric layers: Intima, media and adventitia. The intima contains endothelial cells and smooth muscle cells. It is separated from the media by the internal elastic membrane (elastica interna). The media consists of smooth muscle cells and connective tissue. The adventitia is the outer layer and consists of collagen and elastic fibres. In normal human coronary arteries, the intima thickens with age. In middle age the intima may become diseased by atherosclerotic plaque. Those plaques are formed by an accumulation of lipids, blood, fibrous tissue and calcified deposits and predominantly affect the intimal layer [206]. Figure 1.1 schematically shows typical cross sections of a normal and a diseased coronary vessel.

Over time coronary plaques can lead to a narrowing of the vessel lumen (stenosis). If the blood flow through arteries is thus impaired, the heart muscle is not sufficiently supplied with blood (myocardial ischemia). This may lead to an imbalance between supply and demand of oxygen. The results can be the development of chest pain (angina pectoris). The development of this type of atherosclerosis is generally slow, which leads to stable angina pectoris. It can be treated by medication or interventional techniques.

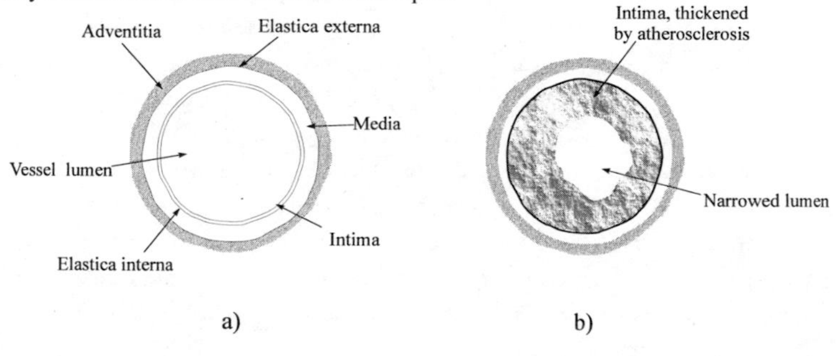

Figure 1.1: Diagram of a normal (a) and a diseased coronary vessel (b)

Rapidly evolving acute coronary events are a more severe problem affecting more than 19 million people world wide each year. A large portion of these patients has no prior symptom [122]. Acute coronary syndromes (unstable angina pectoris, myocardial infarction, and sudden death) are usually caused by an occlusion of the vessel lumen due to thrombosis [159]. This type of coronary thrombosis is caused by so called “vulnerable” plaques [202], which can be divided into three lesion types: Ruptured plaques, eroded plaques and lesions with calcified nodules [201].

Ruptured plaques are the most common lesions and account for more than 60% of all thrombi associated with sudden coronary death or acute myocardial infarction [52, 202]. Rupture prone plaques are characterized by a thin fibrous cap and an underlying lipid-rich, necrotic core [51]. The cap thickness is usually less than 65 μm and is often infiltrated by inflammatory cells (macrophages) [25]. Thus, the thin cap is potentially vulnerable to mechanical stresses and is further destabilized by the inflammation [114].

Plaque erosions occur over lesions rich in smooth muscle cells but do not show cap rupture [201]. They are involved in about 40% of thrombotic sudden coronary deaths [52]. Plaques showing calcified nodules are less frequent. They are characterized by a disrupted fibrous cap and calcified thrombi protruding into the vessel lumen [201].
These aspects show that the composition of an atherosclerotic lesion rather than size and volume or degree of stenosis determines the risk of acute clinical events [103, 139]. In the contrary, coronary occlusion and myocardial infarction most frequently evolve from mild to moderate stenoses [51]. Although only 10-20% of all lesions show vulnerable behavior, they cause 80-90% of the acute clinical events [20]. Thus, evaluating the composition of the vessel wall and its histologic characteristics may be an important step in lesion specific treatment [93].

1.2 Assessment of coronary plaques

The evaluation of morphological and functional characteristics plays an important role in the diagnosis and treatment of vessel diseases. Several invasive and non-invasive methods are currently used for the assessment of atherosclerosis. They can be divided into two groups: Imaging modalities for visualizing plaque morphology and methods for the analysis of functional parameters, such as temperature, mechanical properties or hemodynamic parameters. Besides evaluating plaque size and luminal diameter, some of these techniques have the potential to characterize plaque composition and thus may be able to identify high-risk plaques. Each of these modalities has its advantages and disadvantages, the more important ones are discussed briefly in this section.

1.2.1 Coronary imaging modalities

1.2.1.1 X-ray angiography

Digital angiography is an important imaging modality for the assessment of coronary artery diseases. In this method the lumen of the arteries is visualized by X-ray imaging in conjunction with contrast agents. Coronary angiography is a standard procedure for the assessment of coronary plaques and also for the guidance of interventional procedures. In an invasive catheterization procedure a guiding catheter is inserted into the ostium of a coronary artery and the contrast agent is administered through this catheter. Angiography visualizes the coronary vessel tree in real-time, the resolution is about 0.5 mm [218]. Image processing methods have been developed to quantify vessel and stenosis geometry in digital images[19].

However, the accuracy of this method is limited and strongly depends on the projection angle [194]. X-ray angiography does not image the vessel wall, therefore no information is provided about the composition of atherosclerotic plaques [54].

1.2.1.2 Computed Tomography

Recent technical advances in computed tomography (CT) allow the non-invasive visualization of coronary plaques. In this method, the human body is scanned with X-rays and tomographic images are reconstructed from projections acquired at different angles. Angiography can be performed with electron beam CT (EBCT) and contrast agents [121]. EBCT has been considered as gold standard for the assessment of calcified plaques since the early 1990s [55]. Recently, ultrafast multi-slice CT scanners have been developed with 500 ms rotation time and simultaneous acquisition of four slices. Using electro-cardiogram (ECG) triggering, imaging of the heart can be performed in 30 s with spiral acquisitions [134]. The recent development of 16 slice detectors allows the scan of a complete heart in 20 s, the spatial resolution is in the order of 0.5 mm [61]. During the scan the patient has to hold breath to minimize motion artifacts. Initial results show that multi-slice CT can be used for the non-invasive characterization of coronary lesions. Non-calcified plaques were successfully imaged with multi-slice CT [8]. In a comparative study with intravascular ultrasound, plaque composition could be identified and classified with multi-slice CT [94]. The main limitation of these methods is that coronary imaging can only be performed during certain phases of the heart cycle. This leads to prolonged acquisition times and high radiation dosages.

1.2.1.3 Magnetic resonance imaging

Magnetic resonance imaging (MRI) is a non-invasive modality and has several advantages for medical imaging. No ionizing radiation is used and the injection of a contrast agent is not necessarily required [55]. MRI analyzes the relaxation of proton spins under the influence of strong external magnetic fields. These fields are varied in space and time in order to allow the acquisition of two-dimensional image slices, where the image intensity represents the behavior of proton spins in different tissue regions. With conventional MR systems operating at 1.5 Tesla an in-plane spatial resolution of 300 μm can be achieved [54]. A clinical study demonstrated that vessel lumen and wall morphology can be assessed with MRI [53]. In vitro experiments also showed the potential of MRI for plaque characterization [54]. However, the visualization of coronary arteries with MRI is a challenge due to vessel size and topology as well as cardiac and respiratory motion. The long acquisition times require ECG and respiratory gating. Studies have been performed to visualize coronary arteries during one breath-hold [198], but due to the short acquisition time only a small region of interest could be imaged. Compared to X-ray angiography, MRI currently does not reach equivalent sensitivity and specificity for coronary lesion detection [55].

1.2.1.4 Ultrasound

In medical ultrasound, the tissue is probed with high frequency sound waves in pulse echo mode. Short pulses are emitted that are scattered and reflected by the tissue. The echoes are detected and a gray scale (B-mode) image is formed representing the reflectivity of the tissue.

Imaging of vessels with ultrasound is an established method. Vessels can be examined invasively or from the body surface. The latter is usually applied to large arteries. For instance, transcutaneous high resolution B-mode ultrasound in connection with Doppler flow imaging has become an important modality for the examination of carotid arteries [209]. Transthoracic echocardiography at frequencies around 5 MHz can be used to visualize atherosclerotic plaque in the ascending aorta and the aortic arch [210]. These plaques can also be visualized with transesophageal echocardiography [195]. In this minimally invasive technique an ultrasound probe is placed in the esophagus of the patient. Vessels with smaller diameters require imaging devices with a higher resolution, i.e. higher frequencies. Because the penetration depth is reduced at higher frequencies, non-invasive techniques cannot be applied to image vessels that are located deeper in the body.

Intravascular ultrasound (IVUS) is an invasive modality that images arteries from the inside of the vessel lumen. It is predominantly used for the examination of coronary arteries. A catheter equipped with an ultrasound probe is placed in the arterial system and cross-sectional images of the vessels are obtained in real-time. Figure 1.2 shows a typical IVUS image. The ultrasound frequency currently in use ranges from 20-40 MHz [14]. Two imaging principles have been developed for intravascular use: Single element probes that are mechanically rotated by a flexible shaft and transducers consisting of phased array elements that are electronically switched [13].

IVUS is currently the gold standard for the morphological assessment of coronary artery diseases. It allows the assessment of lumen area as well as size and distribution of coronary plaques [127]. IVUS can also be used for the assessment of plaque composition. By analyzing the spectra of the ultrasound echoes it is possible to discriminate different tissue types and characterize plaque content [124]. Ultrasound strain imaging is also a potential tool for plaque characterization. This method has been shown to be feasible with array transducers in vitro and in animal experiments [39, 40]. The major part of this thesis is dedicated to strain imaging using single element IVUS transducers.

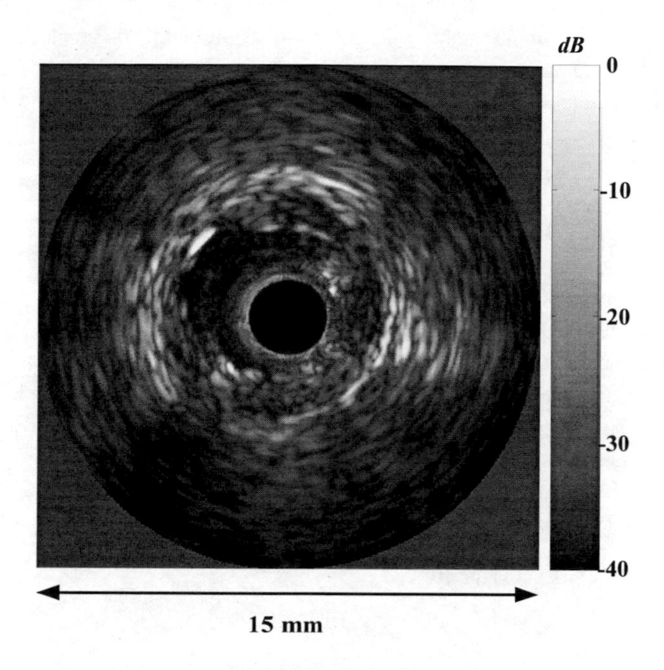

Figure 1.2: Intravascular ultrasound b-mode image

The advantage of IVUS over non-invasive methods is that it gives a detailed cross-sectional view of the coronary wall morphology. The tomographic perspective of IVUS allows visualization of vessels that are difficult to assess with angiography [127]. No ionizing radiation is applied, thus IVUS can be used as a standard application in the catheter lab. A detailed overview of IVUS applications is given in chapter two.

1.2.1.5 Optical coherence tomography

Vascular optical coherence tomography (OCT) is an invasive intravascular imaging modality that allows the acquisition of cross-sectional images at an axial resolution of 10 μm [190]. The physical principles of OCT are similar to those of ultrasound imaging, except that infrared light is used instead of acoustic waves. The tissue is probed by an optical beam and the time delay of light reflected from different tissue segments is measured with an interferometer. In order to obtain a two dimensional image the light beam is scanned across the tissue. For vascular applications a mechanically rotating OCT endoscope was developed, that scans vessels at four revolutions per second [190]. Studies with animal experiments demonstrated that vessel wall imaging is feasible in vivo, with a resolution similar to histopathology [67]. Initial in vitro experiments with human coronary specimens showed that OCT has the potential to discriminate coronary plaque tissue. In a study performed by Yabushita et al. OCT was successfully used to discriminate fibrotic, fibrocalcific and lipid-rich plaques [214]. The main limitation of intravascular OCT is that the vessel wall cannot be imaged in the presence of blood. During in vivo acquisitions the blood flow has to be blocked or the vessel has to be flushed with saline.

1.2.1.6 Angioscopy

Angioscopy images the inner arterial wall surface with light. In an invasive procedure a catheter equipped with fiber optics is inserted into the coronary arteries and video sequences are generated. Angioscopy is used for the investigation of the internal coronary surface and can visualize surface plaque morphology, ulcerations, fissures or tears [80, 111]. It is the only diagnostic technique that provides information on the color of atherosclerotic plaques [98]. Color visualization provides important information about the type of coronary plaque [90]. As with OCT, images cannot be obtained through blood. Therefore the coronary vessel has to be blocked and flushed with saline prior to the acquisition of images. Furthermore, angioscopy only images the wall surface and thus might not be sufficiently sensitive to detect subtle alterations in plaque composition [111].

1.2.2 Functional measurements

1.2.2.1 Thermography

Thermography is an invasive catheter based modality that maps the temperature of coronary plaque formations in a spatially resolved manner. The aim is to characterize plaque tissue and identify vulnerable plaques by evaluating small temperature changes. This method is based on the observation that rupture prone plaques are often infiltrated by inflammatory cells. It was postulated that heat is released by these inflammatory cells and that a temperature difference can be measured on the plaque surface. Temperature sensing devices were constructed to test this hypothesis. Stefanadis et al. constructed a thermography measuring device for coronary applications [183]. A thermistor probe with a temperature accuracy of 0.05°C was mounted on the tip of a catheter. With this device plaque temperature changes were measured in real-time during a catheter pull back. Clinical trials with animal models and patients showed that measurable thermal heterogeneity occurs in diseased arteries, which is assumed to be related to inflammation [184]. A major limitation of this method is the cooling effect of blood flow, which makes temperature differences difficult to measure and leads to an underestimation of plaque temperature. This problem can be overcome by blocking the blood flow with a balloon during temperature acquisition [185]. However, this might not be tolerable for the patient in all cases.

1.2.2.2 Coronary flow velocity measurements

Morphological evaluation often cannot determine if a narrowing of the coronary arteries is flow limiting, which is the main reason for patients' symptoms. In this context the measurement of blood flow velocity is an important tool for the functional assessment of coronary stenoses. Several invasive methods for the measurement of coronary blood flow velocity have been developed for clinical use. For instance, a 12 MHz piezoelectric Doppler ultrasound transducer was integrated in a guide wire, which is inserted into the coronary artery [47]. Another measurement device uses the principle of thermodilution. In this method, a temperature sensor is placed in the distal part of a vessel and a bolus of saline is injected rapidly. The saline flush causes temperature changes, which are recorded during a certain time interval. The mean transit time of the injectant can then be deduced from the temperature curve [34], which in turn gives an estimate for blood flow velocity. The accuracy of both Doppler and thermodilution methods was demonstrated in vivo and in animal models [47, 56]. For clinical use several flow velocity indexes have been proposed. The most common one is coronary flow velocity reserve (CFVR). It is defined as the ratio of maximum flow velocity (induced by medication) to baseline flow velocity, recorded at rest [153]. A low CFVR value indicates that blood flow cannot be sufficiently increased due to the presence of stenoses. However, the main limitation of this method is that it is not lesion specific. By measuring flow velocity alone it is not clear whether the blood flow is diminished by a specific stenosis, by a series of lesions or by a high myocardial resistance. Furthermore, there are no clearly defined normal or cut-off values [153].

1.2.2.3 Coronary pressure measurements

Stenosis severity is determined by the assessment of blood flow, but the evaluation of coronary pressure signals also supplies information about the functional significance of stenoses. By measuring the pressure proximal and distal of a stenosis, lesion severity can be assessed based on pressure differences. During an interventional procedure aortic pressure is routinely measured through a guiding catheter [153]. Thin guiding wires with integrated pressure sensors have been developed, that can measure the pressure distal of a stenosis. If a stenosis significantly reduces the blood flow through the artery, a pressure drop can be observed. Pijls et al. proposed an index called 'fractional flow reserve' (FFR), that evaluates this pressure difference [151]. FFR is defined as the maximal blood flow in the presence of a stenosis in the supplying coronary artery, divided by the theoretical normal maximal flow in the same vessel [152]. A direct relation between coronary pressure and flow can be presumed if the resistances in the coronary circulation are constant, which in theory is the case during maximum blood flow. In that case, pressure measurements theoretically can be used to predict maximum flow and assess functional stenosis severity [151].

FFR is then calculated as the ratio between the mean pressure $\bar{p}_d$ distal of a stenosis and the mean pressure $\bar{p}_a$ proximal of a stenosis:

$$FFR = \frac{\bar{p}_d}{\bar{p}_a} \tag{1.2.1}$$

If no stenosis is present, this ratio equals 1.0. This method is lesion specific [153], which is its main advantage. However, it strongly depends on the state of maximum blood flow, which cannot be achieved in all cases due to microvascular disease [153].

The most accurate way of assessing the functional significance of a stenosis is the determination of its hemodynamic resistance, which can only be accomplished by simultaneous measurement of pressure and flow. A clinically applicable concept for the evaluation of combined pressure and flow velocity measurements is presented in chapter seven.

1.2.3 Summary

As an introduction, this chapter gave a short medical overview of coronary artery diseases. Modalities for the assessment of coronary plaques were presented and advantages of each method were discussed. The main focus was on applications that have already been tested in the clinic and can be used in vivo. Besides imaging plaque morphology, some of these methods can be used to obtain functional information or aim at the detection of vulnerable plaques.

2 Intravascular ultrasound

2.1 Introduction

In medical ultrasound, high frequency sound waves are emitted by a transducer and propagate through the tissue. Along the path, the sound waves are scattered and reflected. Reflections occur at boundaries between homogenous tissue regions that are large compared to the ultrasound wavelength. Tissue elements that are small compared to the wavelength cause diffuse scattering. The waves that are thus propagated back are detected by the same transducer. If the speed of sound in the tissue is known, the location of an echo source can be deduced from the time of flight of the echo signal:

$$r_0 = \frac{c \cdot t_{echo}}{2} \quad (2.1.1)$$

Here, r_0 denotes the distance between transducer and echo source, t_{echo} is the time of flight and c represents the speed of sound. The latter is usually assumed constant for ultrasound image formation.

The amplitude of an echo signal provides information about the reflectivity of the tissue. In amplitude (A-mode) imaging, a single pulse is emitted and the rf-echo signal (A-line) is recorded. The envelope of the A-line is displayed over time, yielding 1-D information about the tissue. The ultrasound pulse travels along a confined directional beam, whose directivity characteristics are determined by the transducer geometry and the signal properties. If the ultrasound beam is translated or rotated, the tissue can be probed in two dimensions. From the demodulated echo signals a gray scale image of the tissue is generated, where the image brightness represents echo amplitude (B-mode imaging). The tissue is probed by either moving the transducer mechanically or by switching the elements of a transducer array. Both principles are applied to intravascular ultrasound imaging and are explained in detail later in this chapter.

2.2 IVUS imaging geometry

Intravascular ultrasound transducers are mounted on the tip of a catheter that is inserted into the vessel under examination. Circular cross-sectional B-mode images are formed with this setup. The imaging geometry referred to throughout this text is displayed in Figure 2.1. The z-direction is the catheter axis which corresponds to the elevational direction of the ultrasound beams, if the transducer aperture is orientated perpendicular to this axis ($\zeta = 90^\circ$). Single element transducers rotate within a sheath. In order to reduce reverberation, the beam angle is slightly tilted ($\zeta > 90^\circ$, see also Figure 2.5). The ultrasound systems display the images in cartesian coordinates (x-y plane). In this work, images are also displayed in polar coordinates, with radial distance r and lateral (circumferential) direction φ. Figure 2.2 exemplarily shows both representations of an IVUS image side by side.

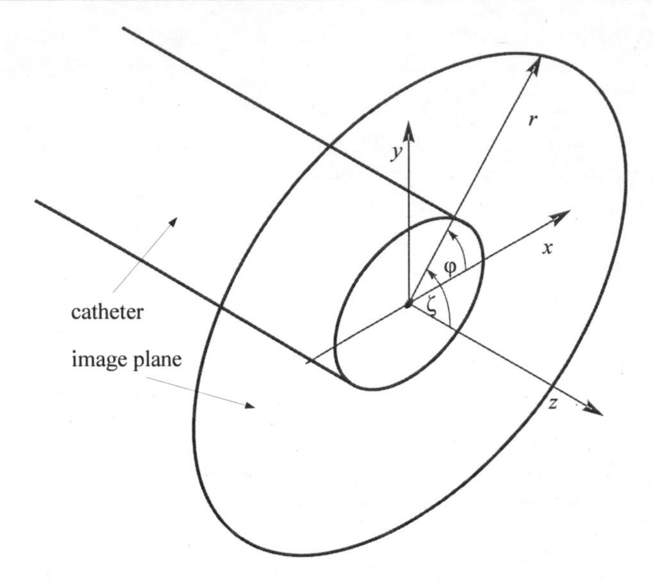

Figure 2.1: Imaging geometry of IVUS

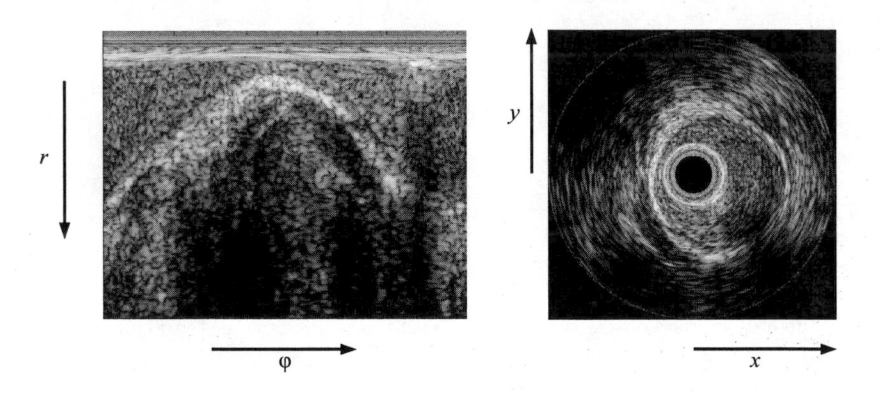

Figure 2.2: Coronary artery in vivo. Left: Polar coordinates (r,φ). Right:Cartesian coordinates (x,y).

2.3 System model

The characteristics of an imaging system are determined by its point spread function (PSF). The point spread function describes the output of the system when imaging an ideal point target and thus defines the spatial resolution [2]. When assuming linearity of the system, the image can be described as a linear transform [78]. In polar coordinates, a system model for the image $b_0(r,\varphi)$ is given by:

$$b_0(r,\varphi)=\int_0^{\infty}\int_0^{2\pi} a(r',\varphi')\cdot h_b(r,\varphi,r',\varphi')\,d\varphi'\,dr' \qquad (2.3.1)$$

In this equation, $a(r,\varphi)$ is the object function representing the distribution of tissue reflectivity. The function $h_b(r,\varphi,r',\varphi')$ is the point spread function. In this representation, the dependency in elevational direction (*z*-direction) is neglected, it is assumed that the ultrasound beam is focused to a thin slice. A further simplification is the assumption of space invariance of the system. In this case, Equation 2.3.1 can be written as a convolution integral [204]:

$$\begin{aligned} b_0(r,\varphi)&=\int_0^{\infty}\int_0^{2\pi} a(r',\varphi')\cdot h_b(r-r',\varphi-\varphi')\,d\varphi'\,dr' \\ &=a(r,\varphi)**h_b(r,\varphi) \end{aligned} \qquad (2.3.2)$$

The point spread function describes how a point scatterer located at $r=r',\varphi=\varphi'$ in the object plane is mapped into the image plane [78]. This becomes clear if the object function is expressed as $a(r,\varphi)=\delta(r-r',\varphi-\varphi')$, where δ denotes the Dirac function. The convolution can then be written as:

$$b(r,\varphi)=\delta(r-r',\varphi-\varphi')**h_b(r,\varphi)=h_b(r-r',\varphi-\varphi') \qquad (2.3.3)$$

Furthermore, in a B-scan system the point spread function is assumed to be separable and can thus be written as:

$$h_b(r-r',\varphi-\varphi')=h_{br}(r-r')\cdot h_{b\varphi}(\varphi-\varphi') \qquad (2.3.4)$$

Here, $h_{br}(r-r')$ characterizes the axial resolution in direction of the ultrasound propagation, while $h_{b\varphi}(\varphi-\varphi')$ represents the lateral resolution in angular direction characterized by the beam width.

2.4 Axial and lateral resolution

The axial resolution in direction of the sound propagation of an ultrasound system is proportional to the bandwidth of the ultrasound pulse received from an ideal point scatterer. The axial resolution can be defined through the minimum distance δ_{ax} at which two ideal point scatterers placed in beam direction are distinguishable. A common measure for this distance is the 'full width half maximum' (FWHM) of an echo received from an ideal point scatterer. This measure is derived by identifying the values of the signal envelope which are half the maximum amplitude. This corresponds to -6dB on a logarithmic scale.

The echo signal received from a point scatterer is often modeled by a sinusoidal pulse with gaussian envelope:

$$x_E(t) = A \cdot e^{-b \cdot t^2} \cdot \sin(\omega_0 t + \varphi); b > 0 \tag{2.4.1}$$

Figure 2.3 shows the gaussian envelopes of the echoes received from two point scatterers with distance δ_{ax}. From the figure it is clear that the two waveforms are not distinguishable if the time delay between the two maxima falls below Δt_{-6dB}.

The axial resolution can therefore be defined as:

$$\delta_{ax} = \frac{1}{2} c \cdot \Delta t_{-6dB} \tag{2.4.2}$$

Figure 2.4 shows a simulated gaussian modulated pulse waveform along with the corresponding spectrum. The FWHM values Δt_{-6dB} and Δf_{-6dB} are reciprocal. For a gaussian modulated pulse the time-bandwidth product results in [203, 211]:

$$\Delta t_{-6dB} \cdot \Delta f_{-6dB} \approx 0.88 \tag{2.4.3}$$

The gaussian modulated pulse is only an approximation to realizable ultrasound signals, where pulses are asymmetric and the time-bandwidth product is higher.

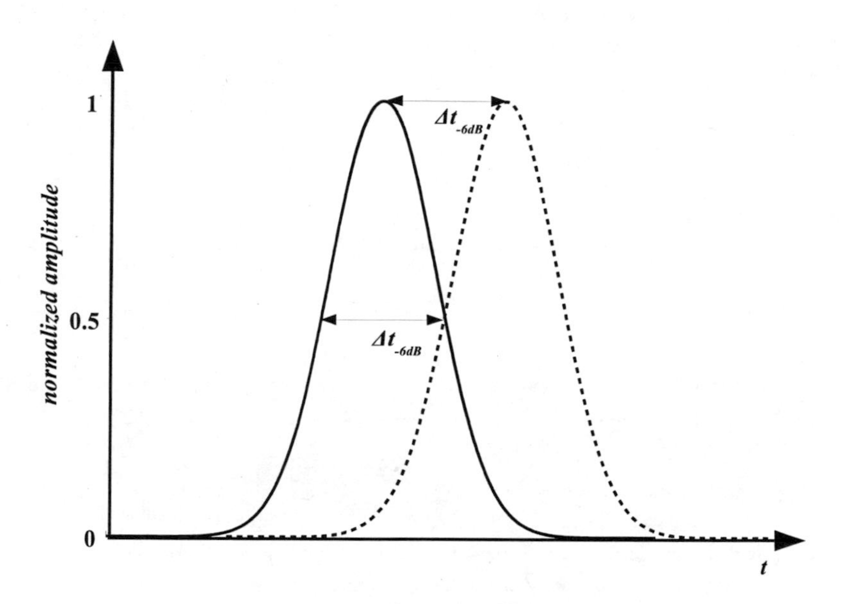

Figure 2.3: Gaussian envelope of echoes received from two point scatterers. The time Δt_{-6dB} corresponds to the FWHM. If the delay between the two maxima falls below Δt_{-6dB}, the echoes will not be distinguishable.

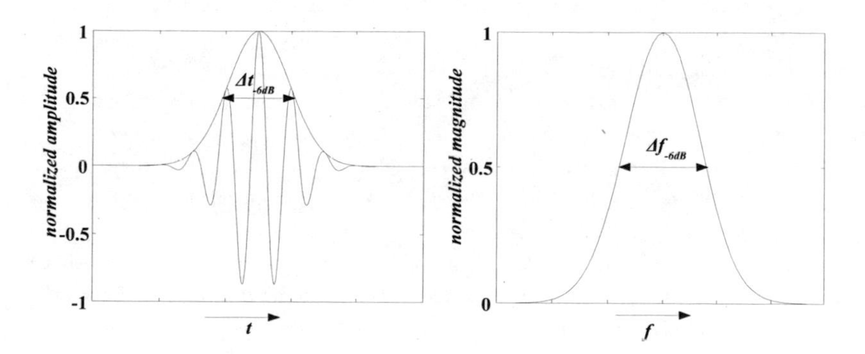

Figure 2.4: Simulated gaussian modulated pulse. Left: Pulse wave form and and envelope. Right: Spectral magnitude.

The lateral resolution of an ultrasound transducer is determined by the lateral beam width. When considering a planar circular transducer, a simplified expression for the lateral resolution δ_{lat} is given by [165,160]:

$$\delta_{lat} \simeq 2.44 \cdot \lambda \cdot \frac{z_F}{D} \tag{2.4.4}$$

Here, z_F denotes the focal length, λ is the wavelength and D denotes the transducer's diameter. The natural focus of such a transducer corresponds to the near field range, which is given by:

$$N = \frac{D^2}{4 \cdot \lambda} \tag{2.4.5}$$

To characterize the lateral resolution it is also common to measure the FWHM of an echo reflected by a point scatterer [64]. Foster et al. define the lateral resolution as [63]:

$$\delta_{lat} = \lambda \cdot \frac{z_F}{D} \tag{2.4.6}$$

Here, δ_{lat} is the width of the beam in lateral direction where the amplitude drops to half the maximum. This expression is valid for unfocused transducers at axial distances beyond the near field range [64]. Except for the factor 2.44 this expression corresponds to Equation 2.4.4.

2.5 Rotating single element transducers

Mechanically rotating intraluminal ultrasound devices have been in use since the 1950s [13]. The early probes have been used for rectal tumor location, transesophageal and intra-cardiac applications as well as imaging of large vessels. In the late 1980s more sophisticated transducer technology and miniaturization allowed the development of intra-coronary imaging devices [161]. There are two categories of single element transducers, which are schematically shown in Figure 2.5. Diagram b) shows a rotating drive shaft with a single element transducer mounted on the tip. The shaft is located in a sheath and connected to an external motor. Diagram a) depicts a setup with a mirror. The static transducer is mounted inside the sheath, the acoustic waves are reflected by the mirror. An image is formed by rotating the mirror. The advantage of this setup is that the static transducer can be connected with wires, while a collector ring has to be used for connecting the rotating transducer. For acoustic coupling purposes the sheath has to be filled with water in both cases.

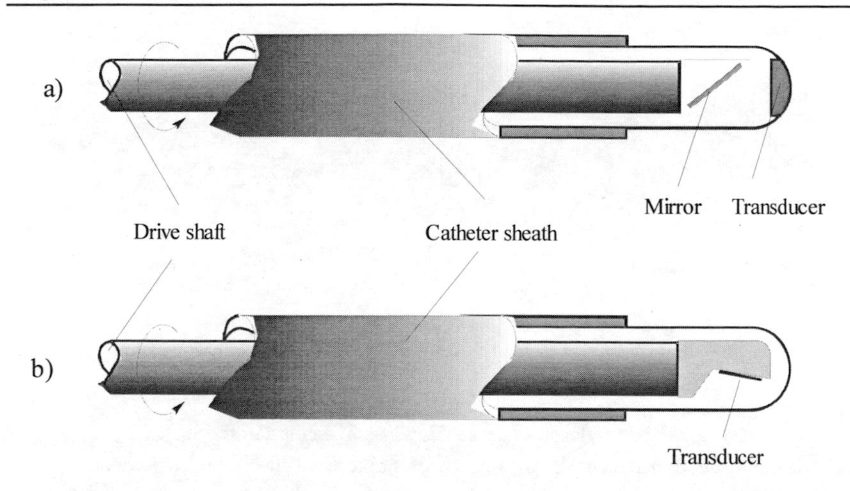

Figure 2.5: Principles of rotating transducers. a): static transducer with rotating mirror. b): rotating single element transducer.

In clinical use the rotating transducers have prevailed. Transducers with 30 MHz and 40 MHz center frequencies are currently commercially available. The outer catheter sheath diameters are 1.06 mm and 1.0 mm, respectively. Figure 2.6 shows a photograph of a 40 MHz transducer mounted on the tip of a drive shaft. The main advantage of single element transducers over the solid state array technology is the use of higher frequencies, which enhances image resolution. The latter currently operate at 20 MHz, higher frequencies would require further transducer miniaturization and more complex focusing techniques. A drawback of the single element transducers is their fixed focus. While the array technology described later in this chapter allows dynamic focusing over depth, the focus of the single element transducer is determined by its geometry and the frequency in use. Another limitation of single element systems is the non-ideal mechanical behavior. Due to friction the rotation speed varies, which causes non-uniform rotational distortion (NURD). This behavior can be a severe limitation, especially for correlation based signal processing. The effects of NURD are investigated in detail in chapter 5.4.

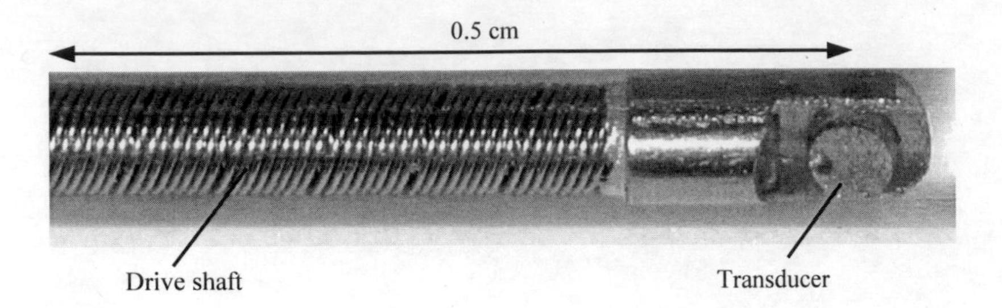

Figure 2.6: 40 MHz single element transducer

2.6 Array transducers

Array transducers were introduced in the 1970s and now belong to the standard technology in medical ultrasound. They consist of a group of single transducer elements which are small compared to the transducer dimensions and have no significant directivity in lateral direction [96]. An active aperture for recording an A-line is formed by a subgroup of elements. The active aperture is translated by switching the single elements electronically, thus a B-scan is formed. In elevational direction, conventional array transducers have a fixed focus. Usually, all elements of an active aperture simultaneously transmit a pulse and the echoes are recorded by each individual element. The advantage of this procedure over single element transducers is the possibility of dynamic receive focusing. This is done by delaying the recorded echo signals according to the time of flight from a desired focus point, followed by summation. This technology also allows electronic beam steering by delaying the transmitted pulses according to the desired direction [96]. Due to the use of single elements the active aperture is spatially sampled, which introduces additional constraints regarding the array geometry. As in classical sampling theory, undersampling has to be avoided. If the distance between the elements (pitch) is too large, grating lobes occur due to undersampling of the wave field [2]. Grating lobes are avoided for steered ultrasound beams if the element pitch d is smaller than half the minimum wavelength λ_{min} of the echo signal:

$$d < \frac{\lambda_{min}}{2}; \quad \lambda_{min} = \frac{c}{f_{max}} \qquad (2.6.1)$$

In this equation, c denotes the speed of sound and f_{max} is the highest frequency of the echo signal spectrum.

In conventional ultrasound imaging linear or curved array transducers are used. In order to obtain a cross-sectional image from within a vessel, IVUS requires a circular array that covers 360°. In the early 1970s Bom et al. constructed the first circular phased array transducer for intracardiac imaging [13] operating at 5.6 MHz. The array had an outer diameter of 3.2 mm and consisted of 32 elements.

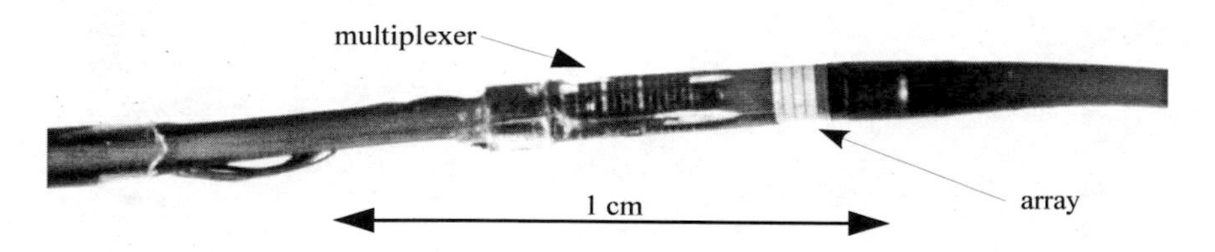

Figure 2.7: 20 MHz array transducer.

In the late 1980s a 32 element intravascular array transducer was constructed [126]. The elements were distributed evenly over the circumference of a circle with 0.9 mm radius, resulting in a 2.3-λ element pitch [130]. This device was further refined to an array with 0.6 mm radius and 1.5-λ pitch [132]. As described above, this element pitch leads to significant grating lobes. This problem was overcome with a modified acquisition scheme that synthesizes a fully sampled aperture function by multiple firings [132]. In this scheme, two firings are made at each position, one in a monostatic mode and a second one in a bistatic mode with a neighboring element. For side lobe reduction, optimal reconstruction filters were developed.

The current state of the art is a 64 element array with 0.6 mm radius and 0.75-λ pitch, Figure 2.7 shows a photo of such a catheter. It operates at 20 MHz with a fractional bandwidth of about 35%. [133]. In contrast to conventional arrays which use all elements of an aperture in transmit mode, there is only one single transmit element and an independent receiving element at each firing. The advantage is that no complex wiring and circuitry for parallel beam forming is required. A multiplexer is integrated into the catheter tip for element switching. Furthermore, both transmit and receive apertures can be dynamically focused [133], since the signals from all single element transmit/receive combinations are recorded. Such an array is schematically shown in Figure 2.8. An active aperture is formed by 14 elements. Beams are formed radially with the aperture centered around it, as indicated by the dotted line. All transmit/receive combinations within the aperture are used for reconstruction. The reconstructed signal at each depth location is formed by coherent summation, which is exemplarily sketched for location P_0. In order to synthesize a complete image, the aperture is switched around the circumference in steps of one element, thus $64 \cdot 14 = 896$ signals are recorded. From this data set, 512 equally spaced beams are reconstructed for image formation. The reconstruction is described in more detail in chapter 4.2.

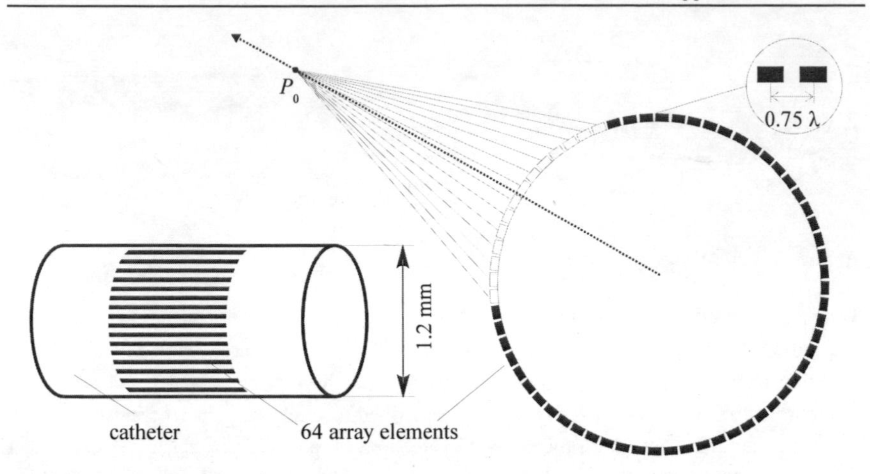

Figure 2.8: 64 element circular array. The active aperture consists of 14 elements, the element pitch is 0.75 λ. Beams are formed radially by coherent summation.

2.7 Intravascular Doppler measurements

Measuring blood flow velocities with ultrasound is a clinically established method. Blood contains erythrocytes, leucocytes, platelet and plasma, where the predominant scatterers of acoustic waves are the erythrocytes (red blood cells) [196]. When an ultrasonic wave is scattered back from a moving target, the echo signals' frequency will be shifted due to the Doppler effect [46]. The Doppler equation in ultrasound relates this frequency shift f_d to the blood flow velocity v by the following equation [2]:

$$f_d = 2 f_0 \frac{v \cdot \cos(\Theta)}{c} \tag{2.7.1}$$

Here, f_0 is the frequency of the transmitted ultrasound signal, Θ denotes the angle between ultrasound beam and blood velocity direction and c is the speed of sound. This equation implies that a velocity component parallel to the ultrasound beam is required in order to measure velocities with this method.

Blood velocities can be either measured with continuous wave (CW) ultrasound Doppler or with pulsed wave (PW) Doppler. In CW mode, an ultrasound wave is continuously emitted by a transducer, the echoes are received by a second transducer. The drawback of this method is that no range information can be obtained. This can be overcome with PW mode Doppler, which allows the measurement of velocities within a selected region. In PW mode, pulses are emitted and received repeatedly by the same transducer at a certain pulse repetition frequency (PRF). However, since the Doppler signal is sampled at each pulse transmission with sampling frequency PRF, an upper blood velocity limit exists which is governed by the

Shannon sampling theorem [2]. If the Doppler frequency shift f_d exceeds half the pulse repetition frequency, undesired frequency aliasing occurs. Thus, the following limit applies for alias free velocity measurements, where T_{PRF} denotes the time between the transmission of two pulses:

$$f_d < \frac{1}{2 \cdot T_{PRF}} \tag{2.7.2}$$

In order to measure higher blood flow velocities, the pulse repetition frequency has to be increased. This again poses a limit on penetration depth, since T_{PRF} cannot be smaller than the time of flight of the ultrasound wave reflected from a desired location. If the blood flow velocities are expected to be high, CW mode Doppler should be preferred, since there is no limit on maximum velocity with this method.

Catheter based intravascular Doppler transducers were constructed as early as the 1960s [13]. Both CW and PW intraluminal transducers have been described. Since the velocity can only be measured parallel to the ultrasound beam with Doppler methods, forward looking transducer elements (z-direction in Figure 2.1) were mounted on the catheter tips.

Presently available IVUS Doppler catheters transmit signals in PW mode. They operate at frequencies of 12-15 MHz at a gated depth of 4-5 mm. Spectrum analysis is performed using the Fast Fourier Transform (FFT) [136]. Short time FFTs are continuously calculated and the Doppler spectra are displayed over time as a gray scale image. From the spectra an instantaneous peak flow velocity (IPV) is derived, which is the basis for the blood flow velocity measurements presented in chapter 7.

2.8 Summary

This chapter described basic principles and the current technology of intravascular ultrasound. The imaging geometry was described and a system model for IVUS was presented along with definitions for lateral and axial resolution. Furthermore, the state of the art in catheter technology was outlined with advantages and disadvantages of single element transducers versus array technology. The chapter concluded with an introduction to intravascular Doppler measurements and instrumentation.

3 Strain imaging with intravascular ultrasound

3.1 Introduction

The development of diseases often involves a change in the mechanical behavior of biological tissue. Physicians routinely use digital palpation for diagnosis of diseases such as cancer or ulceration. However, this method is user dependent and often not accurate. Therefore, the assessment of mechanical properties of tissue with ultrasound became a research topic of major interest in recent years. The main goal of this approach is the visualization of tissue elasticity. For this task the tissue is deformed and simultaneously scanned with ultrasound. The mechanical behavior of the tissue is then estimated from the ultrasound data and visualized. For this procedure the application of a mechanical stimulus is required. The methods developed for this task can be divided into two groups. The first group contains approaches that apply low frequency vibrations to the tissue. Inhomogeneities of tissue stiffness cause a disturbance in vibration patterns, which are analyzed with ultrasonic Doppler methods [69, 138, 215]. In the second group of methods a quasi-static compression is applied to the tissue. The tissue is slowly compressed and ultrasound images are acquired during compression. Regions with different elastic moduli show different levels of tissue displacement and strain, which can be estimated from two or more ultrasound image frames [77, 131, 135]. Several algorithms have been developed to estimate displacement and strain in one and two dimensions either from ultrasound rf-data or demodulated data. These approaches comprise displacement estimates with ultrasound speckle tracking or block matching techniques [11, 131], correlation based algorithms [135], and optical flow algorithms [207]. Usually, the displacement is estimated first, the strain is then calculated as the first derivative of the displacement [85, 200]. This approach was introduced by Ophir et al. [135] and termed 'Elastography'. Other approaches calculate the axial strain along the A-lines directly by adaptively stretching the post compression A-lines [21, 199]. Several groups also developed methods for the reconstruction of the elastic moduli of tissue based on the estimated shift or strain [84, 177, 187].

The methods for the evaluation of mechanical properties of vessel walls with IVUS mostly fall into the second category, because the generation and evaluation of vibration patterns in vessels is hardly feasible in a clinical environment. Thus, a quasi-static compression is applied to the vessel wall and the resulting displacement and strain distribution is estimated from the ultrasound data. Strain imaging with intravascular ultrasound poses specific problems that are not encountered in other applications. In conventional non-invasive strain imaging, the ultrasound transducer is hand held or fixed in an experimental setup. The required tissue compression can thus be controlled and decorrelation due to lateral or out of plane motion can be minimized. Apart from that, the transducer surface is always in contact with the examined tissue and can be used as a reference point with zero displacement. This is not the case with IVUS, where the transducer is located inside the vessel without constriction. The tissue compression cannot be controlled, the source of compression can only be pressure variations due to pulsatile blood flow [42] or a compliant balloon, which is inserted into the vessel [31]. However, the latter approach requires the complete blocking of the vessel, which is hardly tolerable for the patient. Without a balloon, the transducer can move freely within the vessel. This causes several artifacts, which will be pointed out later in this chapter. Since the transducer is not in contact with the vessel, segmentation of the vessel wall is also required to obtain accurate strain imaging results.

Several research groups developed algorithms for the measurement of displacement and strain in vessel walls with IVUS. O'Donnell et al. proposed a Fourier based speckle tracking algorithm for the measurement of arterial wall motion in two dimensions [129]. This approach evaluates signal phase shifts that occur due to tissue displacement. Experiments were performed with vessel mimicking phantoms [174, 175] and with vessel specimens ex vivo [31], using intravascular array transducers. The tissue was compressed with a compliant balloon inserted into the vessel lumen. Ryan et al. constructed a prototype intravascular imaging system [162]. The setup comprised a single element transducer operating at 42 MHz and a rotating mirror. Radial vessel wall motion was analyzed by cross correlating corresponding rf-beams. Motion in two dimensions was also analyzed based on demodulated images by applying a 2-D cross correlation function [163, 164].

Talhami and coworkers developed a strain imaging technique based on the evaluation of spectral features of recorded video images [189]. This method assumes that compression of the tissue results in a time scaling of the signals, which according to the Fourier theorem of scaling also causes a scale change of the spectra. By determining spectral peak locations they derived a mean strain value for each line of the image. The advantage of this approach is that any scanner with a video output can be used for data acquisition. However, the low resolution only allows to calculate a mean strain value for each angle and strain changes in depth cannot be resolved.

De Korte et al. assessed radial tissue displacement and strain with one dimensional cross correlation analysis based on rf A-lines. In vitro experiments were performed with vessel phantoms and excised human arteries using 30 MHz single element transducers [35, 36] or commercially available 64 element intravascular array transducers [39]. The feasibility of this approach was verified in clinical studies with animal models [41] and during human coronary interventions [42]. In these studies deformation was applied by natural variation of the intracoronary blood pressure. Data sets acquired during end diastole were used for evaluation, since image correlation was highest and catheter motion minimal. The same group developed a procedure they termed “ultrasonic palpation” [27]. In this technique tissue strain is measured only in a thin region close to the lumen boundary. This method was reported to be robust and suitable for further real-time applications [27, 48].

Brusseau et al. developed an algorithm that estimates radial strain from IVUS rf-data. In contrast to the previous methods, the strain is calculated directly from a set of ultrasound A-lines by iteratively stretching the post compression signal [21, 22]. In vitro experiments with phantoms and excised carotid artery specimens demonstrated the feasibility of this technique.

Intravascular strain imaging based on video data was investigated by Wan and coworkers [207]. This method uses log-compressed and scan-converted (cartesian) images for motion estimation, which is performed with optical flow algorithms based on the methods proposed by Horn and Schunck [79]. The advantage of this approach is that video data are easy to obtain. However, the low image resolution and errors introduced by scan conversion degrade the accuracy of this method.

3.2 Stress and strain in arteries

The mechanical properties of arteries depend on the composition of the vessel wall and the surrounding tissue. Arteries consist of three layers. They contain smooth muscle cells, elastin and collagen fibers [6]. Therefore, the arterial tissue is an inhomogeneous and anisotropic material. Mechanical properties of arterial walls have been investigated in vitro and in vivo [6, 76]. In animal experiments stress-strain relations have been derived from pressure measurements and changes in vessel diameter recorded over several cardiac cycles [5, 6]. In these experiments intravascular pressure was measured with a microtransducer and the vessel diameter was continuously recorded with an ultrasound transmission sonomicrometer. Stress and strain were calculated from pressure and diameter measurements by using linear elastic theory and assuming an ideal medium for the vessel wall. A nonlinear behavior was shown for the stress-strain relationship in the physiological range of pressure. At low pressure values during diastole a nearly linear elastic behavior was observed, caused mainly by elastic fibers. At higher pressures during systole the relationship became nonlinear due to the contribution of collagen fibers and smooth muscle cells. This nonlinear behavior has to be kept in mind when analyzing the elastic behavior of arteries over a wide range of pressures.

In the case of small deformations however, a linear stress-strain relationship can be assumed. It appears feasible to apply a simplified model in this case and describe the vessel as a linear elastic tube. In conjunction with strain imaging this approximation can be justified by the fact that only data acquired during diastole is used for evaluation, because heart motion is minimal during this phase. The applied strain is small, in the order of 1-3%. With this simplification it is possible to analyze the displacements and strains in a pressurized vessel. This is important for understanding the mechanisms and artifacts of IVUS strain imaging. The elastic tube is assumed to be a homogeneous, isotropic thick walled cylinder as outlined in Figure 3.1. A complete elastic solution for this geometry is given in [4]. This problem can be described by three stress-strain equations (3.2.1), along with three strain-displacement equations (3.2.2).

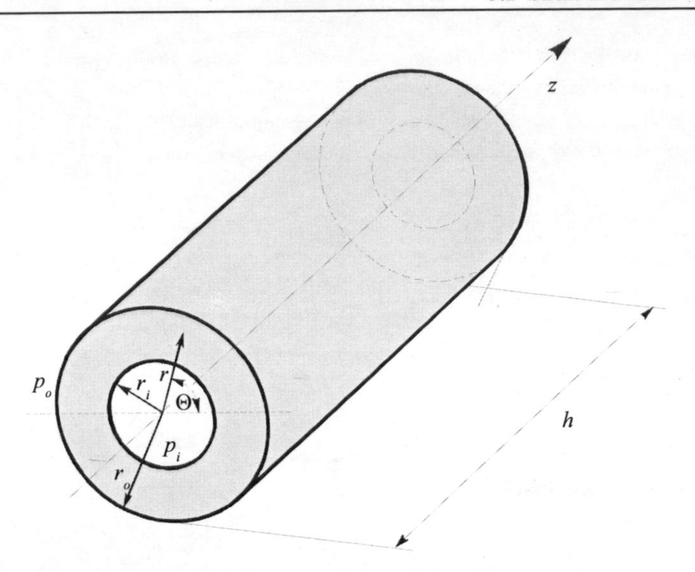

Figure 3.1: The vessel is modeled as a thick walled cylinder model with inner radius r_i, outer radius r_o and longitudinal length h. The inner pressure is p_i, the outer pressure p_o.

$$\epsilon_r = \frac{1}{E}[\sigma_r - \nu(\sigma_\theta + \sigma_z)]$$

$$\epsilon_\theta = \frac{1}{E}[\sigma_\theta - \nu(\sigma_z + \sigma_r)] \quad (3.2.1)$$

$$\epsilon_z = \frac{1}{E}[\sigma_z - \nu(\sigma_r + \sigma_\theta)]$$

$$\epsilon_r = \frac{du(r)}{dr}; \ \epsilon_\theta = \frac{u(r)}{r}; \ \epsilon_z = \frac{dw(z)}{dz} \quad (3.2.2)$$

Here, $\epsilon_r, \epsilon_\theta, \epsilon_z$ are radial, circumferential and longitudinal strain, respectively. The variable $\sigma_r, \sigma_\theta, \sigma_z$ denote the corresponding stresses. E is the modulus of elasticity, the values u and w represent the radial and longitudinal displacement, respectively. The value ν denotes the Poisson's ratio. Biological tissue is considered incompressible [23, 68] and the Poisson's ratio has a value of $\nu \sim 0.5$ in this case. A solution for the stresses for this geometry is given by [4]:

$$\sigma_r = -\frac{p_i\left[(r_o/r)^2-1\right]+p_o\left[(r_o/r_i)^2-(r_o/r)^2\right]}{(r_o/r_i)^2-1}$$

$$\sigma_\theta = \frac{p_i\left[(r_o/r)^2+1\right]-p_o\left[(r_o/r_i)^2+(r_o/r)^2\right]}{(r_o/r_i)^2-1} \qquad (3.2.3)$$

$$\sigma_z = \sigma_0$$

Here, the longitudinal stress σ_z is constant within the cylinder. If the cylinder is assumed to be constricted in longitudinal direction (plane strain problem), the displacement w and the longitudinal strain vanish [4, 112]:

$$w(z)=0 \rightarrow \epsilon_z = \frac{dw(z)}{dz} = 0 \qquad (3.2.4)$$

From Equations (3.2.1) and (3.2.4) an expression for σ_z can be derived:

$$\sigma_z = \nu(\sigma_r + \sigma_\theta) \qquad (3.2.5)$$

The substitution of (3.2.5) into the equation for ϵ_θ in (3.2.1) results in:

$$\epsilon_\theta = \frac{1}{E}\left[\sigma_\theta(1-\nu^2) - \sigma_r \nu(\nu+1)\right] \qquad (3.2.6)$$

Since the radial displacement can be expressed as $u(r) = r \cdot \epsilon_\theta$, it can be calculated by inserting the expressions for the radial and circumferential stresses from (3.2.3) into (3.2.6):

$$u(r) = \epsilon_\theta \cdot r = A \cdot \left[\frac{r_o^2}{r}(P_i - P_o)(\nu+1) - r\left(P_i - P_o\left(\frac{r_o}{r_i}\right)^2\right)(2\nu^2+\nu-1)\right]$$

$$A = \frac{1}{E\left((r_o/r_i)^2-1\right)} \qquad (3.2.7)$$

According to (3.2.2) the radial strain can be calculated as the first derivative of u.

$$\epsilon_r = \frac{du(r)}{dr} = -A \cdot \left[\frac{r_o^2}{r^2}(P_i - P_o)(\nu+1) + \left(P_i - P_o\left(\frac{r_o}{r_i}\right)^2\right)(2\nu^2+\nu-1)\right] \qquad (3.2.8)$$

Note that the radial displacement in Equation (3.2.7) depends linearly on the pressure difference and has two terms that are proportional to the radius. For nearly incompressible tissue the Poisson's ratio approximates 0.5. In this case the term on the right hand side of Equation (3.2.7) vanishes and the dependency can be written as.

$$u(r) \sim \frac{1}{r} \tag{3.2.9}$$

The radial strain on the other hand decays with $1/r^2$. The term on the right hand side in Equation (3.2.8) is not dependent on r and vanishes as well for incompressible tissue. This behavior has to be taken into account when analyzing strain images of phantoms or blood vessels. Tissue regions located towards the outer wall appear stiffer than those at smaller radii, though the tissue might be homogeneous. In the case of a homogeneous vessel and a centered ultrasound transducer, this influence can be eliminated by multiplication with r^2. In practice, this is often not feasible due to tissue inhomogeneity.

3.3 Strain imaging algorithm

In this work, radial strain is estimated from IVUS rf-data sets acquired before and after compression by using one-dimensional correlation techniques. The calculations are limited to one dimension for computational simplicity. Furthermore, radial strain can be estimated with much higher precision than circumferential strain, since radial displacement occurs in beam direction and rf-data can be used for this task.

The principle of IVUS strain imaging is schematically shown in Figure 3.2. The left diagram shows part of a homogeneous circular vessel with the inner and outer vessel walls located at radius r_0 and r_2, respectively. A small region of interest (ROI) is located at r_1, the pressure inside the lumen is p_0. The right diagram shows the same vessel after increasing the pressure inside the lumen by Δp. The vessel tissue is compressed due to the increase in pressure. The ROI is compressed and at the same time displaced radially by Δr. If the ROI is small compared to the vessel dimensions, the compression inside this region can be neglected in comparison to the displacement Δr. Thus, local tissue displacement can be estimated by tracking the region of interest before and after compression.

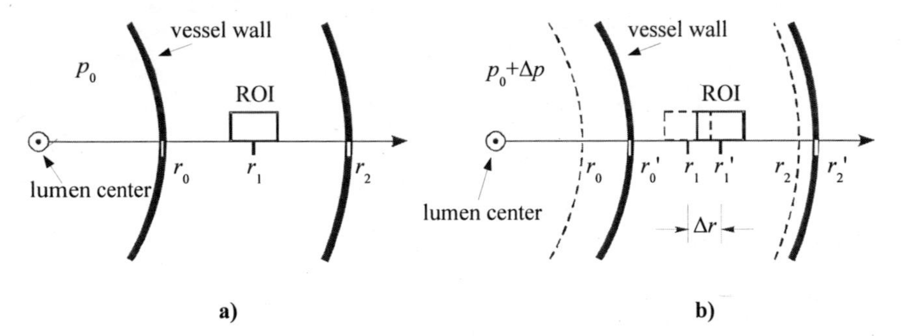

Figure 3.2: Principle of IVUS strain imaging, a) vessel before compression and b) vessel after compression. The region of interest (ROI) is assumed to be radially displaced by Δr.

Assuming that the intravascular ultrasound transducer is located in the lumen center, the radial tissue displacement will be parallel to the ultrasound beam. The displacement can then be estimated from time shifts in ultrasound rf-data, since the tissue displacement Δr is directly related to signal time shift τ by the equation:

$$\tau = 2\frac{\Delta r}{c} \tag{3.3.1}$$

Here, c denotes the speed of sound, which is assumed to be constant in the tissue. In order to obtain local displacement estimates, the signals are divided into overlapping segments and the time shift of the signals before and after compression is determined for each segment. A strain profile can then be calculated as the spatial derivative of the radial displacement.

The algorithm presented in this work estimates the tissue displacement by evaluating phase shifts of corresponding A-lines acquired before and after compression [140, 148].

Let $x_1(t)$ be an ultrasound A-Line acquired without compression and $x_2(t)$ denote an A-Line acquired after compressing the tissue in beam direction. The compression leads to a signal time shift $\tau(t)$. The signals are related by the following equation [110, 149]:

$$x_2(t) = x_1(t+\tau(t)); \text{ with } \tau(t) = \int_0^t \epsilon(t')\,dt' \tag{3.3.2}$$

Here, $\epsilon(t)$ denotes the local compression of the tissue. With the assumption that the compression is constant in a small ROI around a temporal position, the expression for $\tau(t)$ can be written as:

$$\tau(t) = \int_0^t \epsilon_0\,dt' = \epsilon_0 t + t_c \tag{3.3.3}$$

In this equation, ϵ_0 denotes a constant compression factor and t_c is a time constant. A further assumption is that the signal time shift in a small window around the temporal position t_1 is constant. Equation (3.3.2) can then be simplified to:

$$x_2(t) = x_1(t+\tau_1); \text{ with } \tau_1 = \epsilon_0 t_1 + t_c \tag{3.3.4}$$

The time shift τ_1 can be estimated by cross correlating the two A-lines. Under the assumption that $x_1(t)$ and $x_2(t)$ are jointly stationary, the cross correlation function of the two signals is defined as [58]:

$$r_{x_1x_2}(t) = \lim_{T\to\infty} \frac{1}{T} \int_{-T/2}^{T/2} x_1^*(t')\,x_2(t+t')\,dt' \tag{3.3.5}$$

With Equation (3.3.4) it can be shown that $r_{x_1x_2}(t)$ is equivalent to the auto correlation function $r_{x_1x_2}(t)$ shifted by τ_1 :

$$r_{x_1x_2}(t)=\lim_{T\to\infty}\frac{1}{T}\int_{-T/2}^{T/2} x_1^*(t')x_1(t+t'+\tau_1)dt'=r_{x_1x_1}(t+\tau_1) \quad (3.3.6)$$

Since the auto correlation magnitude has a maximum value at zero lag, the cross correlation function consequently has a maximum at $t=-\tau_1$. Therefore, the time shift $-\tau_1$ can be estimated by determination of the maximum cross correlation magnitude [135]. An alternative approach is the evaluation of the signal phase shift, which is introduced by the tissue displacement [131]. The advantage of this approach is the reduced calculation time, which will be shown later in this section.

When considering the corresponding analytic signals [58] $x_{1+}(t)$ and $x_{2+}(t)$, the phase of the complex cross correlation function exhibits a zero at the location of the maximum magnitude:

$$arg(r_{x_{1+}x_{2+}}(-\tau_1))=\varphi(-\tau_1)=0 \quad (3.3.7)$$

Thus, the time shift $-\tau_1$ can be estimated by determining the phase zero.

Figure 3.3 exemplarily shows magnitude and phase of the auto correlation and cross correlation function of simulated analytic ultrasound signals. The auto correlation zero lag is located at $t=0\,\text{s}$. As described in Equation (3.3.4), $x_{2+}(t)$ is a time shifted replica of $x_{1+}(t)$. The time shift between the signals is $\tau_1=10^{-8}\,\text{s}$.
The signals' center frequency is $f_0=20\,\text{MHz}$, which corresponds to a cycle duration of $T_0=5\cdot10^{-8}\,\text{s}$. The magnitude of the cross correlation function exhibits a maximum at $t=-10^{-8}\,\text{s}$, which is accompanied by a phase zero.

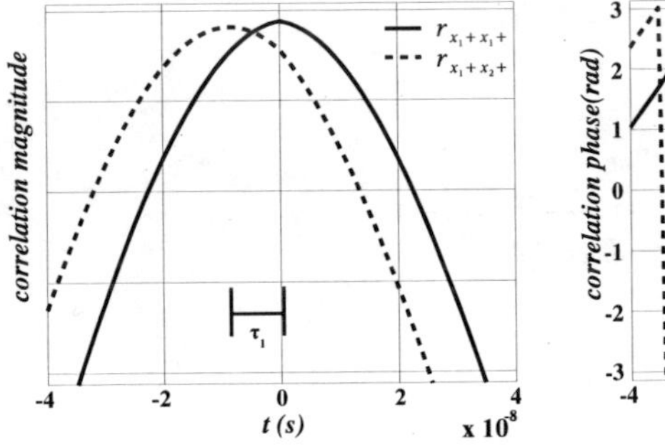

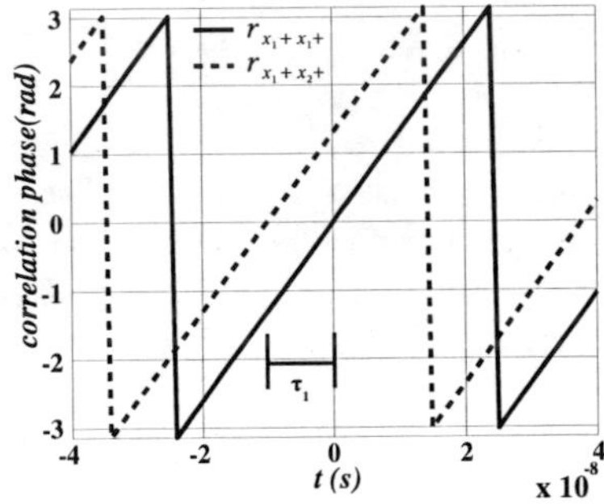

Figure 3.3: Magnitude and phase of the auto- and cross correlation function of analytic signals. The signal shift is smaller than half the signal's cycle duration.

A drawback of the phase evaluation is that aliasing occurs when the time shift is larger than half the signal's cycle duration T_0. This situation is shown in Figure 3.4, where the signal time shift was set to $\tau_1=3\cdot10^{-8}\,\text{s}$. The magnitude of the cross correlation function exhibits a peak at $t=-3\cdot10^{-8}\,\text{s}$ and the time shift can correctly be determined from this maximum. When determining the phase zero, however, due to aliasing the phase shift will be erroneously estimated to be τ_2. As will be shown below, this limitation can be overcome in many cases by determining the cross correlation magnitude once and then adaptively calculating the phase zero in subsequent signal windows while accounting for previous shifts.

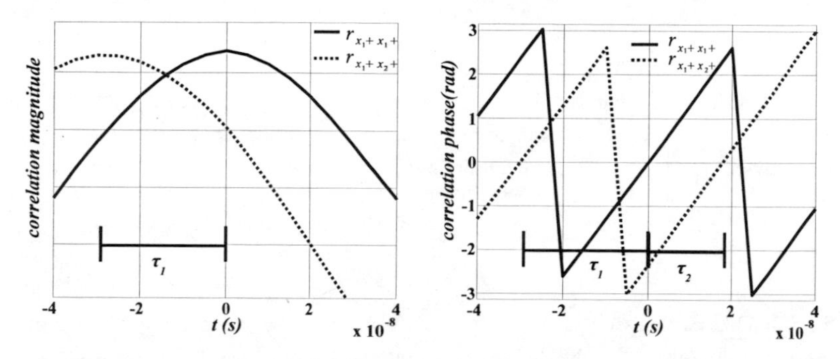

Figure 3.4: Magnitude and phase of the auto- and cross correlation function of analytic signals. Aliasing occurs because the signal shift is larger than half the signal's cycle duration.

A well known method for determining a zero is the Newton's method [17]. The phase zero can be iteratively estimated with the following equation:

$$\tau_{m+1}=\tau_m-\frac{\varphi(\tau_m)}{\varphi'(\tau_m)}\approx\tau_m-\frac{\varphi(\tau_m)}{\omega_0} \tag{3.3.8}$$

The first derivative of the phase $\varphi'(\tau_m)$ is considered to be constant in the vicinity of the phase zero and is replaced by the signal's center frequency ω_0. The advantage of the Newton's method is its fast convergence with only a few iteration steps. The theoretical proof of convergence of this approach was demonstrated in [148].

In practice, the algorithms described above are applied to time-discrete ultrasound signals with finite length that are sampled with the sampling period T_s. The tissue displacements that have to be estimated for strain imaging are often small and the resulting signal shifts can be smaller than the sampling time T_s. For accurate estimates it is therefore necessary to interpolate the signals. For computational simplicity it is desirable to apply simple interpolation algorithms such as nearest neighbor or linear interpolation. In [136] it was shown that an ideal interpolation filter has a rectangular shape in the frequency domain, while the transfer function of a linear interpolation filter can be described by a squared sinc function. If the signals are sampled with a sampling rate close to the Nyquist Rate, the interpolation results will be distorted due to the influence of the sync function. Therefore, linear interpolation should only be applied when the sampling rate is significantly higher than the

Nyquist Rate [136]. An alternative to the application of high sampling rates is the baseband conversion of the ultrasound signals prior to interpolation. The baseband signal is obtained from the analytic signal by a frequency shift of ω_0 :

$$x_b(t)=x_+(t)\mathrm{e}^{-j\omega_0 t} \tag{3.3.9}$$

In baseband representation the spectral power close to the Nyquist Frequency is significantly lower and distortions due to linear interpolation are thus reduced. After the linear interpolation, the frequency shift can be reversed again by multiplication with the term $e^{j\omega_0 t}$. With baseband signals, the Newton iteration in Equation (3.3.8) can thus be written as:

$$\tau_{m+1}=\tau_m-\frac{arg(r_{x_{1b}x_{2b}}(\tau_m)\cdot \mathrm{e}^{j\omega_0\tau_m})}{\omega_0} \tag{3.3.10}$$

In the remainder of this section a formula is derived for the use of the Newton iteration with time-discrete ultrasound signals. The following nomenclature is used for time discrete signals that are obtained from an analog signal $x(t)$ by sampling it at discrete intervals $k\cdot T_s$:

$$x(t)|_{t=kT_s} := x(k) \tag{3.3.11}$$

The signals $x_1(k)$, $x_2(k)$ are divided into overlapping window segments of size N_w. The overlap of the signals is usually chosen in a range from 50% to 75% and is determined by the distance between window segments N_d (see Figure 3.5).

When the pressure inside the vessel lumen is varied, the tissue can be displaced in the order of several wavelengths of the ultrasound signal. In order to avoid aliasing as described in Figure 3.4, the time shifts are estimated in a recursive procedure. First, an initial time shift τ_0 is estimated at the location of the vessel wall by determining the maximum magnitude of the cross correlation function. This is a coarse guess which can be refined by finding the phase zero which is now assumed to be alias free. For this task, the Newton iteration is performed for $m=1..M$ iteration steps. The time shift obtained from this estimate is then used as an initial shift value for the next window segment. This procedure is repeated for all subsequent windows. When considering a window at the location k', the start shift for the Newton iteration is set to the shift result of M Newton iterations of the previous window located at position $k'-N_d$:

$$\tau_{k',0}=\tau_{k'-N_d,M} \tag{3.3.12}$$

The Newton iteration in equation (3.3.10) within the window centered at position k' can then be performed with the following equation:

$$\tau_{k',m}=\tau_{k',m-1}-\frac{1}{\omega_0}\cdot arg\left[e^{j\omega_0\tau_{k',m-1}}\cdot\sum_{\kappa=k'-N_w/2}^{k'+N_w/2}x_{1b}^*\left(\kappa-\frac{\tau_{k',m-1}}{2}\right)x_{2b}\left(\kappa+\frac{\tau_{k',m-1}}{2}\right)\right] \quad (3.3.13)$$

Here, the discrete representation of the cross correlation function is given. The window of interest is centered around position k ($\kappa=k-N_w/2\ ...\ k+N_w/2$). The iteration is performed M times before the window is translated along the signals by the distance N_d.

The tissue strain is calculated as the first derivative of the displacement estimates from consecutive windows. Several groups simply use the difference of displacement estimates to obtain a strain value [26, 135]:

$$\epsilon=\frac{\tau_{k,M}-\tau_{k-N_d,M}}{N_d} \quad (3.3.14)$$

However, this procedure introduces significant errors when the shift estimates exhibit noise. An alternative approach proposed in [85] is the application of a linear regression estimator to a set of N_s displacement estimates. This procedure reduces strain estimate errors and can be efficiently implemented as an FIR filter [140, 149]. Throughout this work, strain was calculated from the shift estimates with such a filter.

With the proposed algorithm tissue displacements can be measured with high accuracy. It was shown that the algorithm reaches the Cramer Rao lower bound (CLRB) for time delay estimations [148]. This bound represents the minimum variance $\sigma^2_{\tau,min}$ achievable in time delay estimations. An expression for this variance is given in [28] for the case of a band -pass signal with a rectangular spectrum:

$$\sigma^2_{\tau,min}=\sigma^2_{CLRB}\simeq\frac{1}{4\pi^2 f_0^2 B\,T\,SNR} \quad (3.3.15)$$

In this expression, f_0 represents the center frequency, B is the signal bandwidth, T is the duration of the observation time ($T=N_w\cdot T_s$) and SNR represents the electronic signal to noise ratio. The equation shows that variance is reduced with increased bandwidth and signal to noise ratio. It also suggests that the observation time should be chosen as high as possible in order to minimize variance. However, in the presence of strain the assumption of a constant time shift only holds for short observation windows. Decorrelation errors occur for larger window sizes in the presence of high tissue strain.

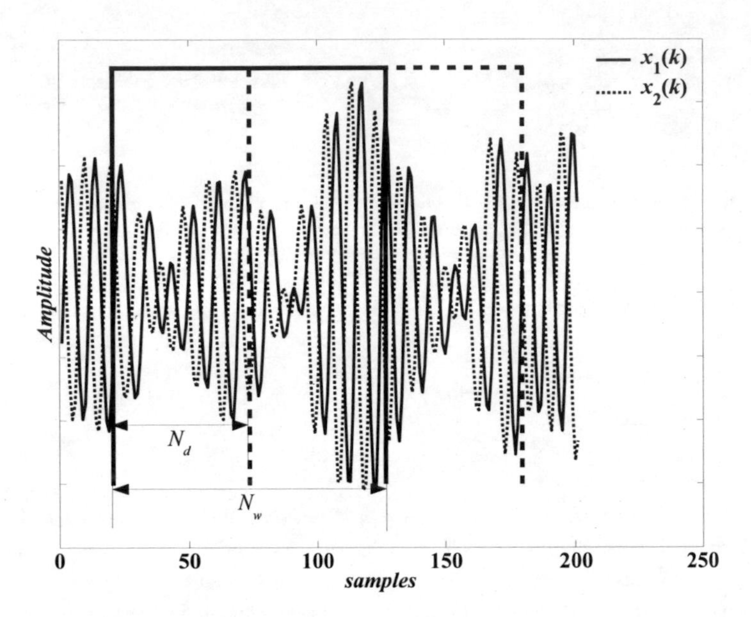

Figure 3.5: A-line pair used for shift estimation. The shift is calculated in windows of size N_w. For each estimate the window is translated along the A-line by N_d samples.

For strain estimation, care has to be taken in the choice of the window sizes and overlap, because there exists a trade-off between resolution and accuracy of the strain estimates. Among other factors, the quality of the strain estimates depends on spatial resolution and the 'elastographic signal to noise ratio' SNR_e [181], which is defined as:

$$SNR_e = \frac{\mu_\epsilon}{\sigma_\epsilon} \tag{3.3.16}$$

Here, μ_ϵ represents the mean value of the estimated strain and σ_ϵ is the standard deviation of the strain. An equation for the strain variance σ_ϵ^2 is given in [28]:

$$\sigma_\epsilon^2 \geq \frac{2\sigma_\tau^2}{T\Delta T} \tag{3.3.17}$$

The value σ_τ^2 represents the time delay estimation variance and $\Delta T = N_d \cdot T_s$ denotes the window distance. According to this equation, strain variance is minimal when $\sigma_\tau^2 = \sigma_{\tau,min}^2$, when the observation windows are long and when the overlap is minimal [10]. On the other hand, short observation windows and a high overlap deliver results with higher resolution [181]. A similar tradeoff exists for the least squares strain estimator. It was shown that such an estimator improves the SNR_e in comparison to the difference in Equation (3.3.14) and rises with increasing window size N_s [85]. However, large window sizes again reduce the resolution.

Finally, the strain variance depends on the amount of strain. In the presence of strain, σ_τ^2 exceeds the lower bound significantly [9], which also leads to a higher strain variance. According to Equation (3.3.16), high strain values on the other hand are required to improve SNR_e.

Therefore, the choice of optimal window sizes is a difficult task which depends on the system parameters, the applied strain and the required resolution. When considering that the strain decreases with the square of the radius (Equation 3.2.8) and that the bandwidth is reduced with increasing depth, a set of window sizes will not be optimal for all regions of an elastogram. Thus, in this work the parameters N_d, N_w and N_s are chosen empirically for the task at hand. Typical values for shift estimation are window sizes from 5 to 20 cycles of the signal's center frequency and 50% to 75% window overlap.

The main advantage of the algorithms is the computational efficiency [149a]. For each step of the Newton iteration the cross correlation function has to be calculated in only one lag, as can be seen in Equation (3.3.13). In [148] it was shown that for a sample data set the mean change in shift estimations $\Delta n = \tau_{k,m} - \tau_{k,m-1}$ is reduced by approximately 20 dB per iteration. Therefore, two to three iteration steps are sufficient in most cases. In the conventional search for the maximum magnitude, the cross correlation function has to be computed in several lags around position k. After that, the signals or the cross correlation function itself have to be interpolated to achieve subsample accuracy. Compared to the proposed algorithm in Equation (3.3.13), a brute force search for the magnitude needed about 20 times more multiplications [148]. Hence, the phase zero search algorithm is suitable for real-time implementations.

3.4 Artifacts in IVUS strain imaging

Due to the special geometry of intravascular ultrasound imaging, several artifacts can occur that degrade morphological measurements as well as tissue strain estimates. Since the ultrasound transducer is not fixed within the coronary vessel, its location and orientation cannot be controlled properly. The heart beats during the image acquisition, which causes motion artifacts. Between two frames the catheter can be translated and/or rotated. Also, during a heart cycle significant longitudinal catheter displacement can occur, sometimes up to 5 mm [3, 43]. In two consecutive IVUS images, those effects lead to in plane and out of plane motion. The ultrasound signal correlation is thus severely degraded and the tissue strain cannot be estimated correctly. Even in the absence of heart motion some artifacts can occur. Systems with mechanically rotating transducers exhibit non-uniform rotational distortions (NURD) [89, 143, 191], which also degrades image correlation. The impact of NURD on strain imaging is examined in chapter 5.4 of this work. Geometric artifacts occur when the imaging catheter is located eccentrically with respect to the longitudinal vessel axis. In addition, it is often tilted forwards or backwards. These effects cause distortions [29, 44, 59, 60], which lead to erroneous measurements and image misinterpretation. Strain imaging results are also influenced by the transducer position. If the vessel is again modeled as a homogeneous isotropic tube, pressurization of the lumen will lead to radial tissue displacement as stated in Equation (3.2.7). If the transducer is centered in the vessel lumen, the direction of displacement will be parallel to the ultrasound beam. In the case of an eccentric or tilted catheter, there is an angle between the ultrasound beam and the displacement. This effect is displayed in Figure 3.6. The left hand side shows a vessel cross section with an eccentric transducer *T*. Due to the angle α only a projection d' of the displacement d is measured, e.g. an underestimation occurs.

Note that in this geometry radial tissue expansion leads to lateral (circumferential) motion in IVUS images, which also degrades image correlation. On the right hand side the case of a tilted catheter is shown. Here radial tissue compression leads to a motion out of the imaging plane due to the angle δ, which again causes decorrelation artifacts. Strain image artifacts caused by catheter eccentricity and tilt were investigated by De Korte et al. [38]. Based on the geometry of the setup they derived analytical expressions for the angles α and δ and the resulting errors in strain estimates. It was shown that the angle α caused by catheter eccentricity is dependent on the penetration depth and the beam direction (represented by the angle θ in Figure 3.6 a). The angle δ was found to be independent of penetration depth, which is obvious in Figure 3.6 b). De Korte et al. corroborated their theoretical results with phantom experiments and showed that systematic strain errors due to the angles α and δ can be corrected. However, the errors introduced due to lateral and out of plane motion cannot be corrected with this method. In the next chapter an alternative approach for the correction of catheter eccentricity for phased array IVUS catheters is presented, where the beam forming is modified so that the beams are parallel to the direction of strain.

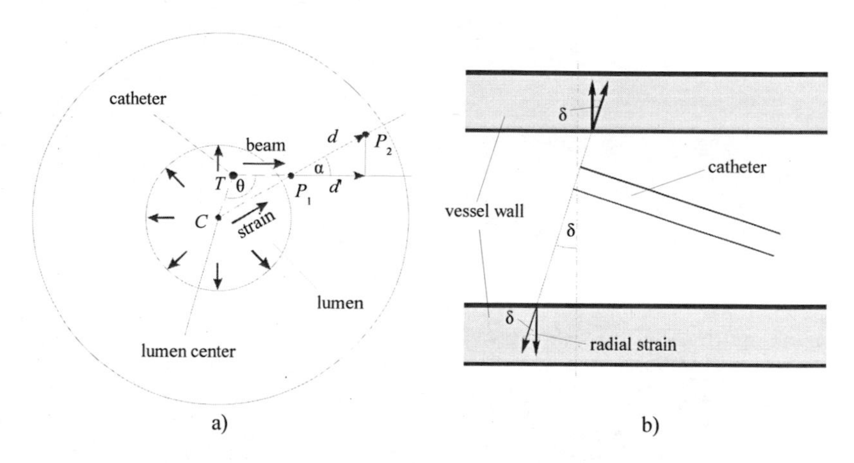

Figure 3.6: Angles between ultrasound beam and direction of strain cause strain image artifacts. a): An eccentric transducer position leads to a depth dependent angle α. b): The angle δ is caused by a catheter tilt with respect to the longitudinal vessel axis.

3.5 Summary

In this chapter the principles, algorithms and limitations of intravascular ultrasound strain imaging were discussed. The application of IVUS shows special geometric properties, therefore the mechanical behavior of vessel walls was recapitulated and illustrated with a simplified cylindric model. It was shown that radial displacement as well as strain are a function of the radial distance, which has to be taken into account when interpreting strain images. Furthermore, the strain imaging algorithm used in this work was explained in detail. It estimates radial tissue displacement and strain by determining the phase zero of complex cross correlation functions of A-lines acquired before and after compression. The algorithm can be implemented efficiently and is real-time capable. It was also shown that the performance of this recursive algorithm depends on an accurate initial shift estimate to avoid phase aliasing, which occurs when the displacement exceeds half a wavelength at the ultrasound signal's center frequency. Finally, as an introduction to the following chapters an overview of artifacts was given that can occur during intravascular ultrasound strain imaging.

4 Strain imaging with array transducers

4.1 Introduction

Array beamforming has become a standard technology for ultrasound applications [2]. This technology is versatile and allows dynamic focusing and beam steering. As in radar processing, synthetic aperture focusing techniques (SAFT) have been widely applied for this task [24, 87 ,216]. IVUS array transducers as described in chapter 2.6 have adopted this technology. Strain imaging with IVUS array transducers has been investigated for several years [35, 37, 41,144]. The main advantage of this technology is the solid state array, thus motion artifacts caused by moving parts of the transducer are absent. However, the frequencies are currently limited to 20 MHz and the required catheter diameters in the order of 1 mm leave little scope for transducer optimization concerning the signal to noise ratio (SNR).

In this chapter, the strain imaging approach described in chapter 3 is applied with IVUS array transducers. First, the beam formation with array transducers is described in more detail. After that, experimental strain imaging results obtained with phantoms are presented. The chapter concludes with a concept for the reduction of strain artifacts based on a modified SAFT beamforming approach [142].

4.2 Synthetic aperture focusing

The ultrasound probe considered in this work is an array transducer as presented in chapter 2.6. For the experimental studies, an ultrasound system (In vision, Jomed/Endosonics, USA) with a custom made analog rf-signal output was available that provided the single channel data before beamforming. A detailed description of the device and the applied synthetic phased array acquisition scheme is given in [133].

The array consists of $N_e=64$ elements. An aperture is synthesized from multiple firings which are acquired consecutively, i.e. only one element transmits at a time. Out of the 64 elements a sub-aperture of $N_A=14$ elements is used to synthesize one beam. Transmit and receive elements are rotated around the transducer, resulting in 896 signals. All signals (transmit and receive) in the sub-aperture are used to reconstruct the image. Thus a circular image is formed with the ultrasound probe in the center. The image consists of $N_b=512$ beams, in this work each line consists of $N_{Samples}=1024$ samples, acquired at a sampling frequency of $f_s=100\,\text{MHz}$. Thus, the image diameter is about 16 mm. Each location in polar image coordinates is described by the radial distance r_i and the angle φ_j with the following conventions (the speed of sound c is assumed to be constant):

$$r_i=0.5\cdot c\cdot i\cdot T_s;\ i=0..N_{Samples}-1 \tag{4.2.1}$$

$$\varphi_j=(j-1)\cdot\frac{2\pi}{N_b};\ j=1..N_b \tag{4.2.2}$$

Image reconstruction can be performed in the time or in the frequency domain [204]. In this work, time domain beamforming by coherent summation was applied as described in [173, 204]. The imaging geometry is shown in Figure 4.1. The highlighted elements form the active aperture. If element m transmits and element n receives an echo from a point scatterer located at position $P(r_i, \varphi_j)$, the wave has traveled the distance:

$$R_{mn}(r_i,\varphi_j)=R_m+R_n=\sqrt{(R_0+r_i)^2+R_0^2-2R_0(R_0+r_i)\cos(\Theta_m-\varphi_j)}+\sqrt{(R_0+r_i)^2+R_0^2-2R_0(R_0+r_i)\cos(\Theta_n-\varphi_j)} \quad (4.2.3)$$

With coherent summation, each echo signal is delayed corresponding to the distance traveled. For a certain position $P(r_i, \varphi_j)$ all signals that are transmitted and received by the elements of the active aperture are delayed and summed up to form the focused beam. The data at a given point will thus be reconstructed by:

$$f(r_i,\varphi_j)=\sum_{n=n_c-N_A/2-1}^{n_c+N_A/2}\sum_{m=n_c-N_A/2-1}^{n_c+N_A/2} W_{mn}\cdot x_{mn}\left(R_{mn}(r_i,\varphi_j)\right) \quad (4.2.4)$$

In this equation, x_{mn} denotes the signal transmitted by element m and received by element n. The value n_c denotes the index of the center element of the active aperture ($n_c=1..64$). Since the array is circular, element indices are wrapped around when exceeding the range of $1..64$. The center element has to be switched depending on the beam angle φ_j and is determined as:

$$n_c=\left\lceil j\frac{N_e}{N_b}\right\rceil;\ j=1..N_b \quad (4.2.5)$$

The function W_{mn} in Equation (4.2.4) is an apodization (weighting) function for sidelobe reduction [204]. An apodization weight is applied to the transmit as well as the receive element, thus the function W_{mn} is the product of two weights:

$$W_{mn}=W_m\cdot W_n \quad (4.2.6)$$

In [173], several apodization functions were analyzed regarding their performance. A triangle windowing function was shown to be a good compromise between side lobe level and resolution and is adopted in this work. The triangle windowing function W_n is given by:

$$W_n=1-\left(\frac{\left|\left(a-\frac{N_A-1}{2}\right)\right|-0.5}{\frac{N_A}{2}}\right);\ 0\leq a<N_A \quad (4.2.7)$$

The windowing function W_m for the transmit aperture is calculated equally.

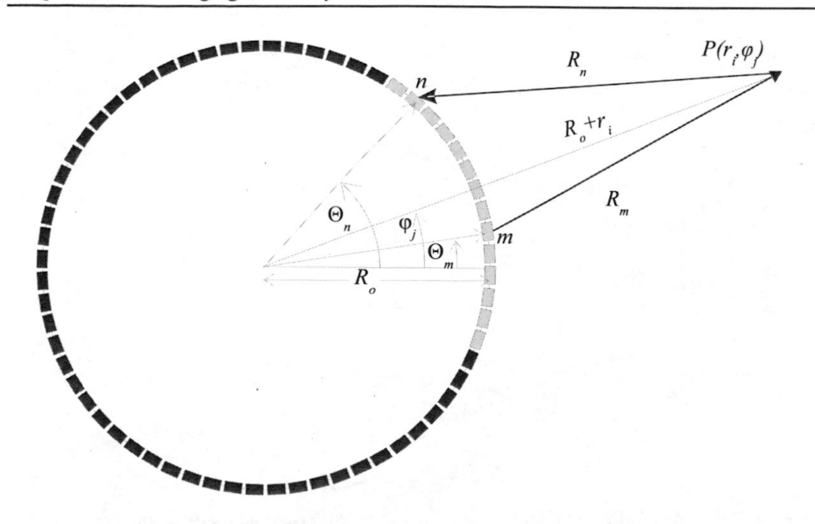

Figure 4.1: SAFT imaging geometry. An active aperture consists of 14 elements, all transmit/receive combinations are used for image reconstruction. The diagram shows an example with element m as transmitter and element n as receiver.

The coherent summation given in Equation (4.2.4) is repeated for all sampling points of the focused A-lines, resulting in a 1024×512 rf-data array. For each data point, the distance traveled by the sound wave according to Equation (4.2.3) has to be calculated for all transmit/receive combinations in a time consuming manner. However, the distances for a specific depth r_i do not change from beam to beam and Equation (4.2.3) can be efficiently implemented with lookup tables.

Figure 4.2 a) exemplarily shows a B-mode image in polar coordinates obtained from simulated data (details of the simulations are given in chapter 4.4). Six point scatterers were placed at different depths and signals from all single channel transmit/receive combinations were simulated. The transmit pulse was simulated as a gaussian pulse with 20 MHz center frequency and 35% fractional bandwidth. The image shows the point scatterer response after coherent summation at a dynamic range of 60 dB. The axial resolution determined by the FWHM of the pulse envelope is $\delta_{ax}=0.1\,\text{mm}$, the lateral FWHM corresponds to 6.3° in angular direction. The lateral resolution increases linearly with the radius, the echo at 2.8 mm depth for instance has a lateral beam width of $\delta_{lat}=0.31\,\text{mm}$. The scatterers close to the transducer surface exhibit side lobe and grating lobe artifacts. The diagram b) displays the beam pattern at 2.8 mm depth. The grating lobes show amplitudes of -43 dB, the sidelobe amplitudes are approximately -35 dB. In comparison to simulation results given in [133], the sidelobe amplitudes are slightly increased, while the grating lobes are reduced. With increasing radius, the grating lobes are beyond the dynamic range and not visible anymore. A detailed description of artifacts and concepts for sidelobe and grating lobe reduction can be found in [99, 132, 173].

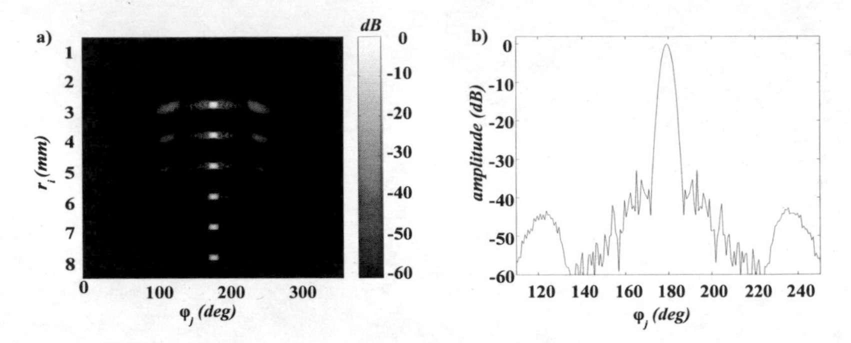

Figure 4.2 : a): reconstructed image of six point scatterers located at different depths (simulated data). b): Beam pattern obtained at the location of the point scatterer closest to the transducer (2.8 mm).

4.3 Phantom experiments

4.3.1 Methods

Phantom experiments were performed in order to verify the SAFT implementation and to investigate the strain imaging performance with the acquired data.

An intravascular ultrasound scanner was used for the experiments in conjunction with 64 element circular array transducers (Endosonics Visions Five 64 F/X) with 20 MHz center frequency. The scanner provided analog, unfocused rf-data from echos of single element transmit/receive operations at a frame rate of $30s^{-1}$. Custom hardware was developed for acquisition control and signal amplification [141, 204]. Based on the trigger signals for each A-line and each image frame obtained from the IVUS system, an output trigger signal was generated to control analog to digital (A/D) conversion. To compensate for depth dependent attenuation, a custom made time gain control (TGC) unit was used. Digitization was performed with an 8 bit A/D converter (Compuscope 8500, Gage Applied, Canada) at a sampling frequency of 100 MHz. A-lines were reconstructed using the synthetic aperture focusing techniques described in the previous section. Vessel phantoms were created from Agar and Polyvinyl Alcohol Cryogel (PVA) [15, 66], respectively. The phantoms were of cylindrical shape, consisting of two layers with different stiffness. With agar phantoms, this difference can be achieved by varying the agar concentration, a range of 1 to 4% concentration in a water solution was used in this study [15]. PVA is a material well suited for constructing vessel mimicking phantoms, because its mechanical properties are similar to those of vessel tissue [65]. It is robust and easy to handle, and can be stored for several months without deterioration. The elasticity of this material can be controlled by the number and duration of freeze-thaw cycles, the material becomes harder with multiple exposure to freezing temperatures [15, 33, 125]. In this work, each freezing cycle lasted for about 10 hours at a temperature of –20° Celsius. Two-layer phantoms were created with an eccentric soft inner layer, which underwent 2 freeze-thaw cycles. For the harder outer layer three cycles were used. Since the scope of this work comprises qualitative analysis only, the elastic moduli of the materials were not determined. In all cases, agar as well as PVA phantoms, silica gel was added as scattering material, because the solutions show low echogenicity. The same concentration of silica gel was used for all materials. Thus, layers of different elasticity show similar echogenicity and cannot be distinguished in B-mode images, but should be clearly identified in the strain images.

The geometries of the two layer phantoms are shown in Figure 4.3. The phantoms have a soft inner layer, which is located eccentrically with respect to the lumen center. A phantom with a highly eccentric circular inner layer is outlined diagram a). This geometry was realized with Agar. The diagram b) shows a phantom that has a slightly eccentric inner layer. A phantom with this geometry was made from PVA. The eccentricity of the inner layer was introduced to distinguish the strain differences of the two layers from the geometry dependent radial strain decay (see chapter 3.2). The diagram c) displays a cylindric phantom structure.

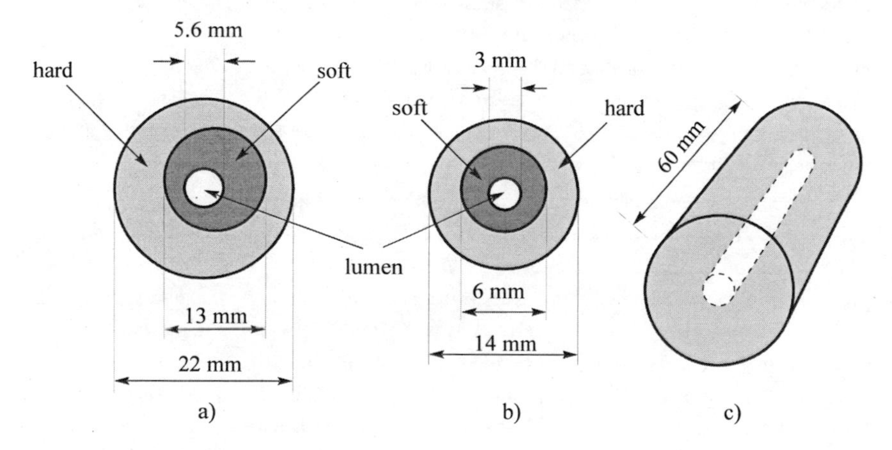

Figure 4.3: Geometry of cylindric two-layer vessel phantoms. a): Circular eccentric soft inner layer (Agar phantom). b): Circular soft inner layer with slight eccentricity (PVA phantom). c) Cylindric structure.

Experiments were performed in a water tank. A cross section of the experimental setup is shown in Figure 5.21. The phantoms were fixed on a mount which was immersed in water for imaging purposes and to prevent dehydration of the phantom material. The phantom lumen was also filled with water. The inner lumen pressure was varied by changing the water level in an attached water column. The catheter was inserted through a watertight sheath and placed in the center of the lumen. For each phantom, a series of images was acquired at different static pressure levels. Strain images were calculated from the acquired rf-data as described in section 3.3. The lumen segmentation required for strain calculation was performed with a threshold algorithm [15].

4.3.2 Results and discussion

In Figure 4.4, the B-mode image acquired with the Agar phantom (Figure 4.3 a)) is displayed along with a radial strain image. The shift between pairs of A-lines was calculated with a window length of 8 wavelengths and 75% overlap, the strain was calculated with a 30 tap linear regression filter. The two layers can hardly be discriminated in the B-mode image alone, whereas in the strain image the different layers can clearly be identified. Compared to the inner layer, the stiffer outer layer shows up as a region of low strain at 6 to 11 o'clock. An overall decrease of the strain towards the outer image regions is also visible. This occurs due to the cylindrical phantom geometry, where the radial strain decreases with the square of the radius. For the shown case, a pressure difference of 1.4 mmHg is applied, which results in a maximum strain of 0.7 %. Figure 4.5 shows images obtained from a PVA phantom with a slight eccentric soft inner layer (Figure 4.3 b)). The shift was calculated with a window length of 8 wavelengths and 75% overlap, the strain was calculated with a 20 tap linear regression filter. In this case, the applied pressure difference was 0.7 mmHg. The eccentricity of the phantom is less prominent than in the case of Figure 4.4, thus it can hardly be seen in the strain images. Overall, phantoms made from PVA proved to be a better suited material for vessel phantoms than Agar. PVA does not break under pressure and can be stored longer than phantoms made from Agar.

Variations of intraluminal pressure differences and subsequent strain calculations showed that local strain can be estimated up to 2.5% [15]. Beyond this point significant decorrelation of the signals occurs and strain images are degraded. This effect is caused by lateral and out of plane motion. Also, at large compressions the speckle patterns in the ultrasound images change, which leads to decorrelation effects as well. Below 2.5% strain, the results show that strain imaging is feasible with the described setup and the applied algorithm, differences in tissue stiffness can be qualitatively distinguished by strain images. For in vivo cases however, limitations apply which have to be taken into consideration. The applied algorithm estimates radial shift and strain. Lateral motion leads to decorrelation effects, which might impose a problem with higher strains or in the presence of heart motion. In order to increase accuracy, the algorithm might have to be extended towards a 2-D estimate. The detection of the inner vessel lumen required for the strain estimation algorithm is done with a threshold algorithm. This is sufficient for phantom experiments, for experiments with vessel specimens or in vivo applications on the other hand a more sophisticated segmentation algorithm is required due to the complex geometrical structure of the vessels.

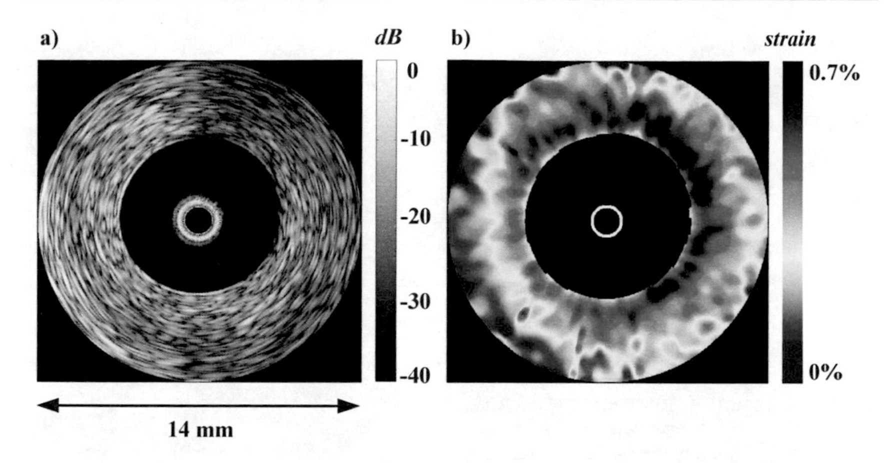

Figure 4.4: B-mode image (a) and corresponding strain image (b) of a two layer Agar phantom with a highly eccentric soft inner layer.

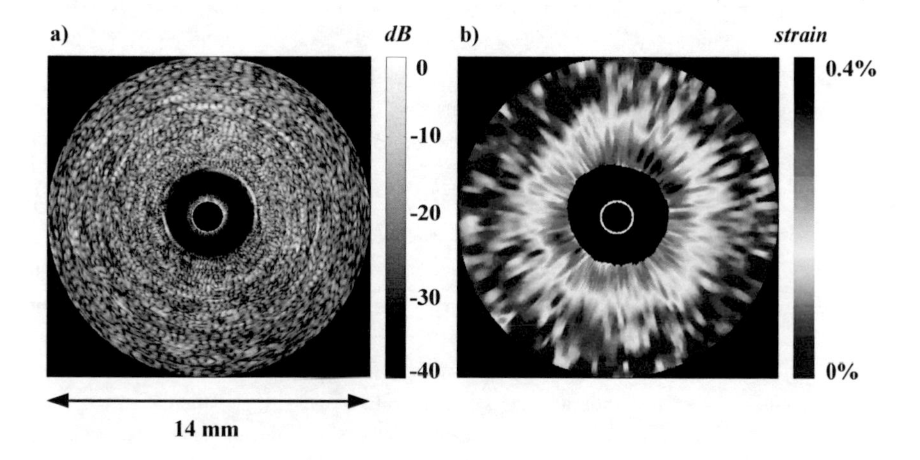

Figure 4.5: B-mode image (a) and corresponding strain image (b) of a two layer PVA phantom with a slightly eccentric soft inner layer.

The applied strain algorithm was shown to be time efficient in other cases [143, 150]. In this application, the signals have to be reconstructed first by coherent summation. In the ultrasound machine this is done by application specific hardware in an optimized way. On a personal computer however, the reconstruction takes several seconds. Alternative concepts, such as described in [204], may speed up the data processing.

4.3.3 Conclusions

The experimental results show that strain imaging is feasible with this setup and the applied algorithms, which is a basis for further clinical trials. For the required detection of the inner phantom boundaries the threshold algorithm performed sufficiently well. Local strain distributions of up to 2.5% can be estimated, at higher strains decorrelation occurs. The proposed algorithm is capable of calculating strain distributions in real-time, but the described setup requires time consuming synthetic aperture image reconstruction, which prevents online imaging. For further studies it would be desirable to have direct access to beamformed rf-data. The single channel data exhibit a poor SNR and the use of a custom made data output is not feasible for a system in clinical use.

4.4 Correction of geometric strain artifacts

Considering a homogeneous vessel with a circular structure, the force that compresses the tissue from within the lumen is normal with respect to the vessel wall and originating from the lumen center. If the ultrasound transducer has an off-center position in the lumen or is not aligned with the vessel axis, there is an angle between force and ultrasound beam. This leads to systematic bias errors in the strain estimate as described in chapter 3.4, since the applied correlation techniques calculate strain in radial beam direction. Moreover, decorrelation due to lateral motion perpendicular to the ultrasound beam degrades the accuracy of the estimates.

These phenomena have been described in detail by De Korte et. al [38]. In their work, they investigated the effects of eccentric and tilted catheter positions and derived a theoretical description of the resulting artifacts. It was also shown that the systematic errors can be corrected with knowledge of the catheter position with respect to the vessel wall. In another study, Shapo et al. [174, 175] addressed the systematic errors due to eccentric catheter positions. They developed a strain imaging method that references all computations to the geometric center of the vessel lumen by a linear 2-D image transformation. Combined with a geometric correction, this method compensates for the described systematic error as well as for catheter motion during image acquisitions.

Both methods estimate the tissue displacement by first evaluating the acquired data and then performing a correction of the systematic errors caused by misalignments. To minimize the mentioned decorrelation caused by lateral motion it would be desirable to realign the ultrasound beams with the compression force rather than apply a correction algorithm on the displacement estimates afterwards.

In this chapter an alternative approach for the correction of strain artifacts is presented, where the ultrasound beams are refocused parallel to the compressing force [142]. Thus, artifacts due to eccentric catheter positions are compensated. Catheter tilt is not considered in this study. This procedure does not require additional geometric correction, since the angle between force and strain is eliminated before beam formation.

The approach is based on SAFT. Conventionally, ultrasound beams are formed in radial direction with respect to the catheter center. But the concept of phased array imaging allows beam steering by varying signal delays, thus beams in different directions can be formed. The beams do not have to originate from the catheter center. Therefore, in this work the focusing technique is modified by forming beams with a direction originating from the lumen's geometric center rather than from the catheter center, provided that the location of the lumen center is known (in a simple circular geometry, the position of the probe with respect to the lumen center can be estimated from the lumen contour in the B-mode images, see Figure 4.6).

The feasibility of this approach was investigated with various simulations. Vessel tissue at different pressure levels was simulated. Intravascular ultrasound rf-data were simulated with different eccentric catheter positions. Strain images were calculated using the algorithm described in chapter 3.3. Results with and without the described correction are compared to evaluate the method's performance.

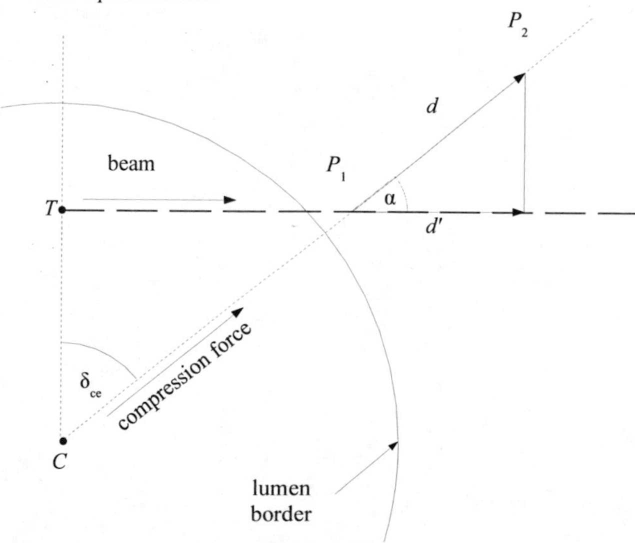

Figure 4.6: Strain projection error due to catheter eccentricity.

4.4.1 Modified Synthetic Aperture Focusing

The case of an eccentric catheter position is depicted in Figure 4.6. The compressing force originates from the lumen center C, the tissue element at location P_1 is displaced by the distance d to location P_2 due to tissue compression. The ultrasound beam formed by the transducer T has an angle α with respect to the force direction. Only the projection d' of the true displacement d is estimated.

This leads to an estimation error that varies with depth and depends on the angle δ_{ce} between direction of force and catheter eccentricity, as shown by the following equation:

$$\alpha = \arcsin\left(\frac{|\overrightarrow{CT}|}{|\overrightarrow{TP_1}|}\sin(\delta_{ce})\right) \quad (4.4.1)$$

The angle α decreases with depth and vanishes with a centered catheter and for angles $\delta_{ce} = n \cdot \pi$. Another source of errors is the lateral motion perpendicular to the ultrasound beam, which is proportional to $\sin(\alpha)$, when considering radial tissue motion due to compression from within the lumen. This motion leads to decorrelation of rf-signals and degrades the performance of the radial shift estimation. Therefore, it is expected that beams formed parallel to the compression force improve the accuracy of strain estimation.

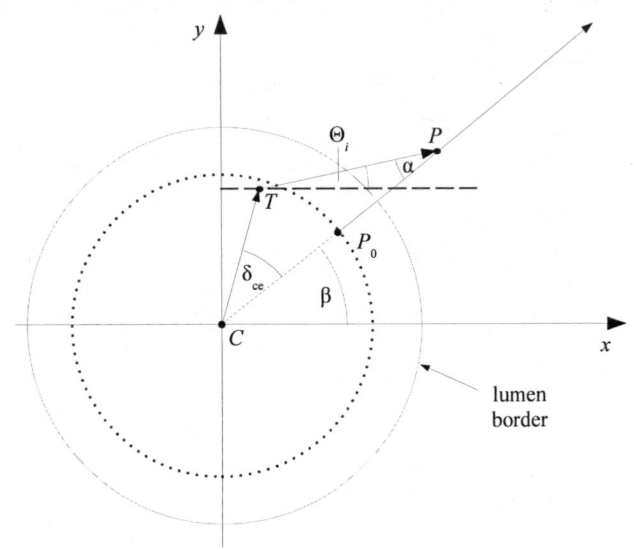

Figure 4.7: Imaging geometry of the modified beam forming approach.

The imaging geometry is shown in Figure 4.7. The coordinate system is centered in the lumen center C. The aim is to form a beam in radial direction with respect to the lumen center C. In order to reconstruct a signal at position P (position vector $\vec{P} = (x_p, y_p)$), the appropriate 14 element aperture of the catheter and the corresponding depth have to be selected (denoted by the angle Θ_i and distance $|\overrightarrow{TP}|$). Given a known catheter center position T (position vector $\vec{T} = (x_t, y_t)$), these values can be calculated by vector analysis:

$$|\overrightarrow{TP}| = \sqrt{(x_p - x_t)^2 + (y_p - y_t)^2} \quad (4.4.2)$$

$$\Theta_i = arg\{(x_p - x_t) + j(y_p - y_t)\} \tag{4.4.3}$$

After calculation of $|\overrightarrow{TP}|$ and Θ_i the previously described coherent summation can be performed with all elements in the aperture. Note that the distance $|\overrightarrow{TP}|$ corresponds to the range $R_0 + r_i$ in Figure 4.1. This procedure is repeated for all desired beam locations, with ultrasound beams formed in radial direction with respect to the lumen center C. Note that the beams do not start in the lumen center, since some would have to cross the imaging catheter. Inside a circle around the lumen center with the radius $|\vec{T}| + R_0$ (dashed circle in Figure 4.7) no data are reconstructed. R_0 is the catheter radius as shown in Figure 4.1. The ultrasound beam outlined in Figure 4.7 for instance starts at position P_0. In practice, this radius should be chosen larger than $|\vec{T}| + R_0$. On the one hand, reconstruction close to the catheter surface corrupts beam formation due to near field artifacts. On the other hand, the ultrasound probe shows a ring-down artifact which produces undesired results at the catheter location.

4.4.2 Simulations

The simulation of ultrasound data for strain imaging applications consists of two parts: First, vessels are simulated with different states of mechanical compression. Second, ultrasound rf-data are generated at each compression state.

In this work, two dimensional simulations were performed. Cylindrical vessel phantoms were simulated by placing randomly distributed point scatterers within the vessel boundaries. The vessels were considered homogeneous, the inner diameter was 5.8 mm, the outer 16.9 mm. The vessels were assumed as a lossless medium, i.e. tissue dependent attenuation was not considered. A compression of 1.3% was simulated by shifting the point scatterer locations according to the applied compression. Only radial shift proportional to $1/r$ was considered in this work. The cylindrical phantoms were simulated with 0%, 20%, 40% and 60% transducer eccentricity with respect to the lumen radius.

The simulation of rf-data was performed by generating A-lines based on the echo response of point scatterers. A circular array with 1.2 mm diameter and 64 elements was simulated. The center frequency was 20 MHz, the element spacing about 0.75λ. Approximately 500.000 scatterers were placed randomly within the phantom boundaries. The smallest resolution cell had an approximate size of 0.032 mm^2, the area of the phantom was 197.9 mm^2. Thus, each resolution cell contained at least 80 scatterers, which is considered a sufficient number for fully developed speckle [205]. The scatterer reflectivity was distributed normally.

In the simulation process it is assumed that a wave is emitted from a transmitting element m. This wave is reflected by a point scatterer and reaches the receiving element n. This procedure has to be repeated for all transmit/receive combinations and all scatterers in the field of view of the elements. 896 signals with 1024 samples at a sampling frequency of 100 MHz were simulated. For reasonable calculation times the number of reconstructed beams was reduced and images consisting of 64 A-lines were reconstructed.

4.4.3 Results and discussion

The Figures 4.8 to 4.11 show the results for different catheter eccentricities. B-mode images over a dynamic range of 40 dB and corresponding strain images of the simulated data are displayed. The radial shift and strain was estimated from A-line pairs before and after compression as described in chapter 3.3. In order to calculate the strain from the estimated time shift, a 20 tap linear regression filter was used. Due to the filter ringing, strain directly at the lumen-tissue boundary cannot be calculated. This part of the image was blanked out and the lumen area in the strain image appears slightly larger. The maximum strain was 1.3% at the tissue boundary, decreasing quadratically with the radius. The strain is displayed in a range from 0.4% to 1.3%. Figure 4.8 shows the results with a centric catheter position, as expected the strain is homogeneous in angular direction. The catheter position is shown as a white circle.

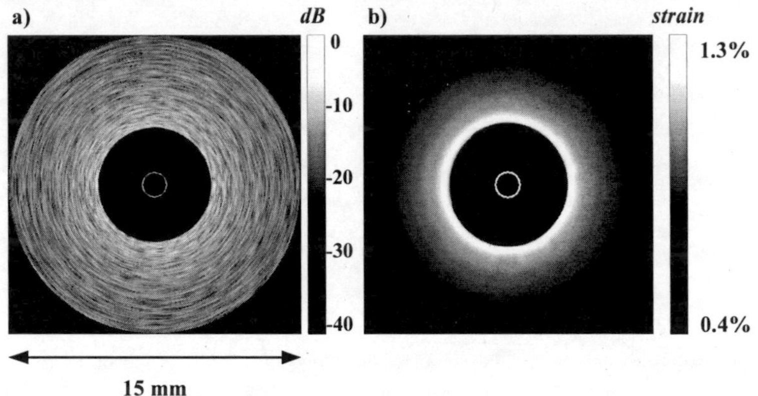

Figure 4.8: B-mode image with 40 dB dynamic range (a) and strain image (b) of a simulated phantom. The transducer (white circle) is centered in the phantom lumen.

The Figures 4.9 to 4.11 display results of the conventional and the modified beamforming approach at different eccentricities. Part a) displays images with conventional beamforming. The beams originate from the catheter center. Part b) displays images reconstructed with the modified beamforming scheme. The beams originate from the lumen center, which is marked by the white circle. Note that this is not the real catheter position. A 20% catheter eccentricity is displayed in Figure 4.9. The strain projection error is hardly visible when comparing the two strain images. Figure 4.10 shows results with 40% catheter eccentricity. The B-mode image in part a) shows a higher brightness in the phantom area closest to the transducer. This effect occurs due to the spherical nature of the simulated waves, whose pressure field decreases reciprocally with the radius [97]. Strain in direction of the catheter shift (6 and 12 o'clock) is still estimated correctly, because the beams are aligned with the direction of compression force. The strain at 3 and 9 o'clock in the strain image of part a) is lower due to the projection error. The overall strain variations are higher than in the centric case, which is caused by lateral decorrelation. Figure 4.10 b) shows a B-mode image centered about the lumen center. The phantom area at 6 o'clock is closest to the real transducer position and again exhibits an increased brightness in the B-mode image, because the radial decrease in amplitude was not compensated in the modified beamforming scheme. The strain projection artifact is eliminated in the bottom strain image, because beams are formed parallel to the compression force. The strain distribution is homogeneous again and angle independent, though with higher strain variations than in the centric case.

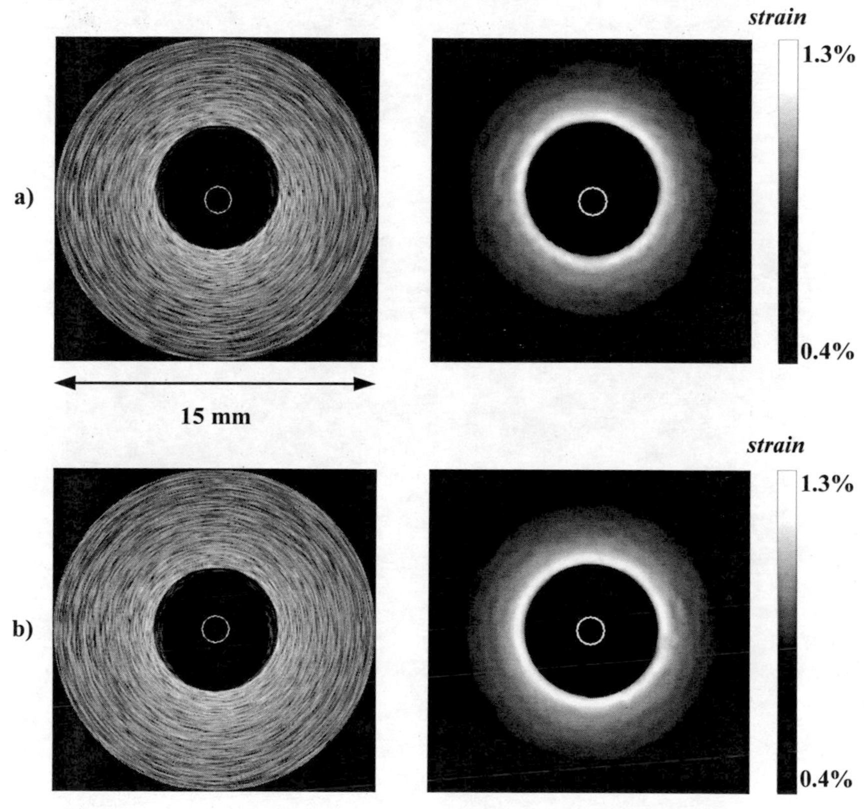

Figure 4.9: B-mode images with 40 dB dynamic range (left) and strain images (right) of a simulated phantom with 20% transducer eccentricity. a): Beams originate from the catheter center, the white circle represents the actual transducer position. b): Beams originate from the lumen center .

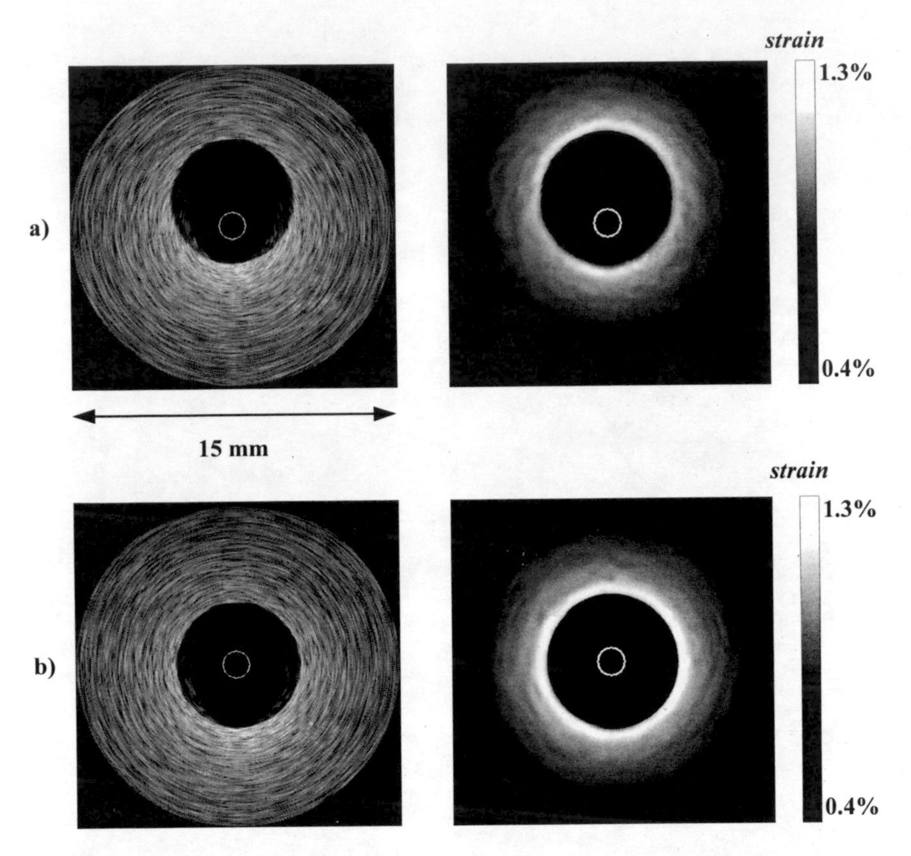

Figure 4.10: B-mode images with 40 dB dynamic range (left) and strain images (right) of a simulated phantom with 40% transducer eccentricity. a): Beams originate from the catheter center, the white circle represents the actual transducer position. b): Beams originate from the lumen center .

Figure 4.11 displays images with 60% catheter eccentricity. The transducer is located close to the lumen border and near field artifacts are visible in both B-mode images around 6 o'clock. The strain projection error is clearly visible in the strain image of part a) as areas of lower strain at 3 and 9 o'clock with respect to the catheter. The plots at the bottom illustrate that the modified beamforming approach can successfully be applied for artifact correction at 60%

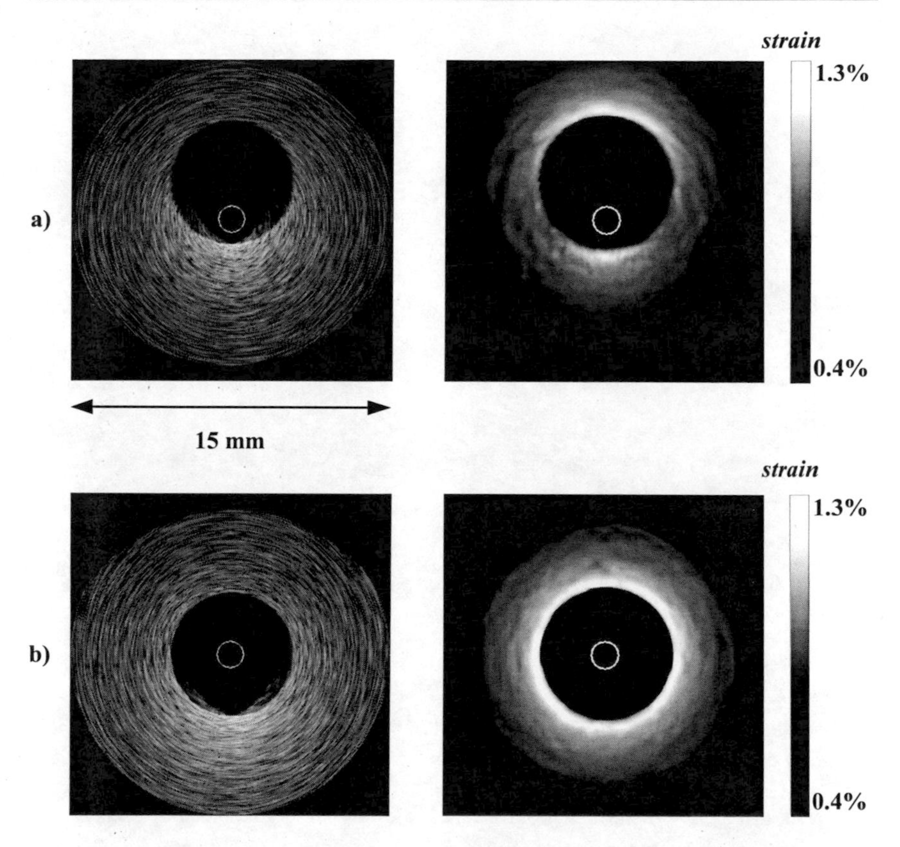

Figure 4.11: B-mode images with 40 dB dynamic range (left) and strain images (right) of a simulated phantom with 60% transducer eccentricity. a): Beams originate from the catheter center, the white circle represents the actual transducer position. b): Beams originate from the lumen center .

eccentricity. The strain projection error is eliminated and the strain is angle independent again. Eccentricities beyond 60% were not considered, because the transducer would be too close to the phantom surface, as can be seen in the B-mode image of part a).

In Figure 4.12, the strain close to the tissue boundary is shown versus the beam angle. An angle of 0° corresponds with the shift direction of the catheter ($\delta = 0$ in Figure 4.6). Plot a) shows the results with traditional beamforming. The strain projection error is prominent around 90° and 270°, where the strain reaches its minimum. The error vanishes at 0° and 180° because the compression force and the ultrasound beams are parallel. Plot b) displays the results with the modified beamforming approach. The systematic strain projection error is corrected by forming beams parallel to the compression force.

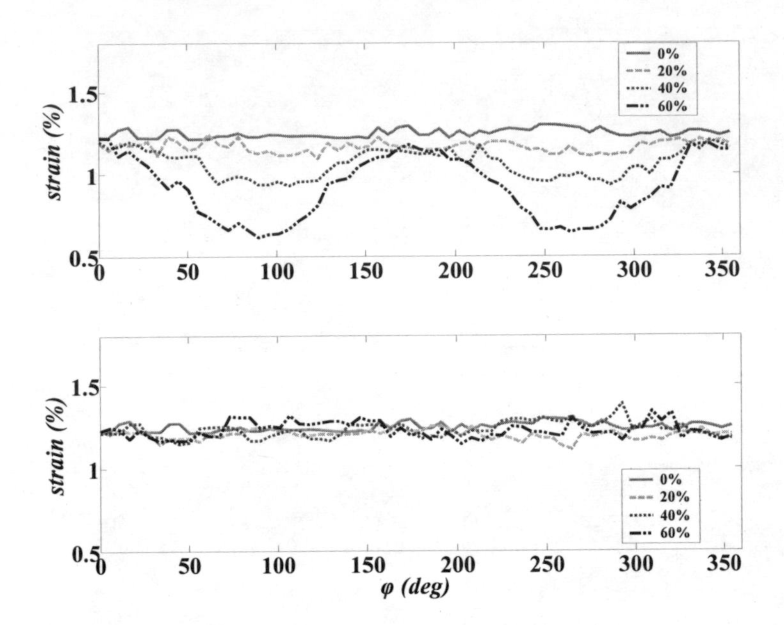

Figure 4.12: Strain at the lumen boundary for 0%, 20%, 40% and 60% eccentricity plotted versus the beam angle. a): No correction was applied, a strain projection error occurs. b): Beams were formed originating from the lumen center, the projection error is eliminated.

The plots in Figure 4.12 show that the strain projection artifact is already present at 20% eccentricity. A visual inspection of the strain images suggests that this artifact becomes prominent only beyond 20%. At 60% eccentricity, the artifact can definitely lead to misinterpretation of the strain image. However, the correction of this artifact is successful in all cases. The proposed modified beamforming approach also has the potential to compensate catheter motion between the acquisitions before and after compression, since the lumen center is used as a point of origin for the beams at all times.

4.4.4 Conclusions

The simulations illustrate that a strain projection artifact occurs with catheter eccentricity. Beyond 20% eccentricity this artifact may lead to misinterpretation. If no correction is applied, images with high catheter eccentricities have to be excluded from strain analysis.

The modified beamforming approach successfully eliminates the projection artifact. However, when applying this beamforming scheme with ultrasound data of coronary arteries, various effects have to be taken into account. First, vessel tissue is highly inhomogeneous and even in a circular structure the expansion due to pressure changes is usually not uniform.

Thus, the geometric center will not be the origin of force for all angular directions. Second, the typical vessel lumen is not circular and the lumen border has to be detected with high accuracy in order to determine the center of gravity. As shown in chapter 6, accurate segmentation is often difficult in vivo. Using an angioplasty balloon with an integrated transducer as proposed in [31, 174] might overcome some of these problems. Due to the balloon inflation the lumen expansion is more uniform. A balloon also facilitates the contour detection, because its surface can be used as a reference. However, expanding a balloon in the coronary arteries and thus blocking the blood flow completely for imaging purposes is usually not tolerable.

4.5 Summary

This chapter described several aspects of strain imaging with intravascular array transducers. The specific synthetic aperture beamforming approach for IVUS array transducers was explained in detail. Phantom experiments and simulations showed that strain imaging is feasible with data reconstructed from single channel acquisitions. The simulations illustrated that an eccentric catheter position leads to systematic errors in the strain estimate with intravascular strain imaging. A method for correcting these artifacts was presented using a modified synthetic aperture focusing technique. The results show that this method is feasible for correcting systematic strain errors due to an eccentric catheter position.

5 Strain imaging with rotating single element transducers

5.1 Introduction

Rotating single element transducers have been used for the examination of coronary arteries since the late 1980s. They allow high resolution imaging with frequencies of up to 40 MHz.

This chapter describes several aspects of IVUS strain imaging with single element transducers. First, transducer characteristics are presented and axial and lateral resolution are determined. The experimental setup for data acquisition is also described along with custom developed hardware for data acquisition. The setup allows continuous data recording and calculation of strain images during the data acquisition. After that, the influence of non-uniform rotational distortion (NURD) on image correlation is assessed. This effect can severely degrade strain estimation results because ultrasound beams are misaligned. For the reduction of NURD artifacts, concepts for beam realignment are presented and verified experimentally. Furthermore, the performance of the algorithms presented in chapter 3.3 in conjunction with single element transducers is investigated in vitro. Experimental results from phantoms and excised human arteries are presented. The chapter concludes with strain imaging results from an in vivo study.

5.2 Transducer characteristics

5.2.1 Axial resolution

In order to determine the axial resolution of the ultrasound system used for the experiments, echoes from an acrylic plate acting as an ideal reflector were recorded. Acquisitions were performed in a tank containing de-ionized water. The plate was aligned perpendicular to the ultrasound beam's elevational direction. The plate was positioned at different depths and the distance with the maximum echo amplitude was determined. Figure 5.1 shows a typical B-mode image of an acrylic plate. The plate echo is visible at as a bright spot at 1.5 mm depth. The echoes around 3 mm depth occur due to multiple reflections. Since the transducer is rotating during the acquisition, an echo is only visible in a limited number of A-lines. The A-line with maximum echo amplitude of each frame was selected for the analysis. The Figures 5.2 and 5.3 show the wave forms and power spectra of echoes acquired with a 30 MHz transducer (UltraCross 3.2, Boston Scientific Scimed, USA) and a 40 MHz transducer (Atlantis SR, Boston Scientific Scimed, USA), respectively. The axial resolution δ_{ax} was determined from the signal envelope as the FWHM-value according to Equation (2.4.2).

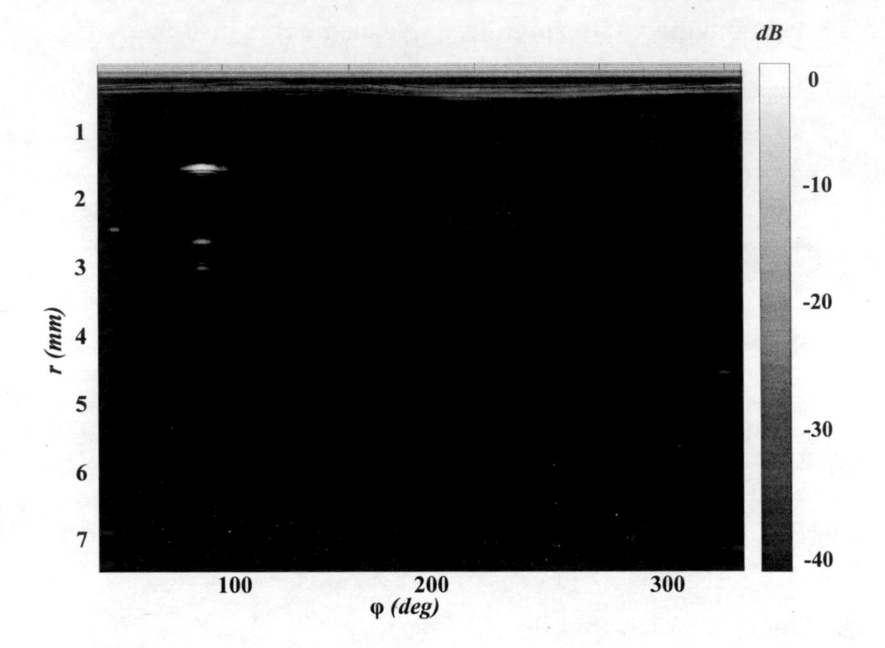

Figure 5.1: B-mode image in polar coordinates recorded with a 40 MHz transducer. The echo of the acrylic plate is visible at 1.5 mm depth.

The results of the measurements are summarized in Table 5.1. The values were averaged over five measurements at a constant plate location.

	δ_{ax}	f_c	Δf_{-6dB}	$\Delta t_{-6dB} \cdot \Delta f_{-6dB}$	Fractional bandwidth
30 MHz transducer	64 μm	27.4 MHz	10.7 MHz	0.91	39%
40 MHz transducer	56 μm	38.1 MHz	14.4 MHz	1.08	38%

Table 5.1: Results of measurements with an acrylic plate.

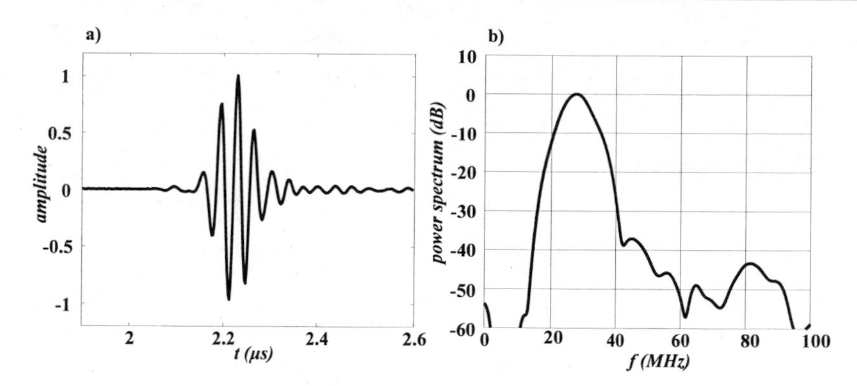

Figure 5.2: Echo from an acrylic plate acquired with a 30 MHz transducer. a): Pulse wave form. b): Logarithmic power spectrum.

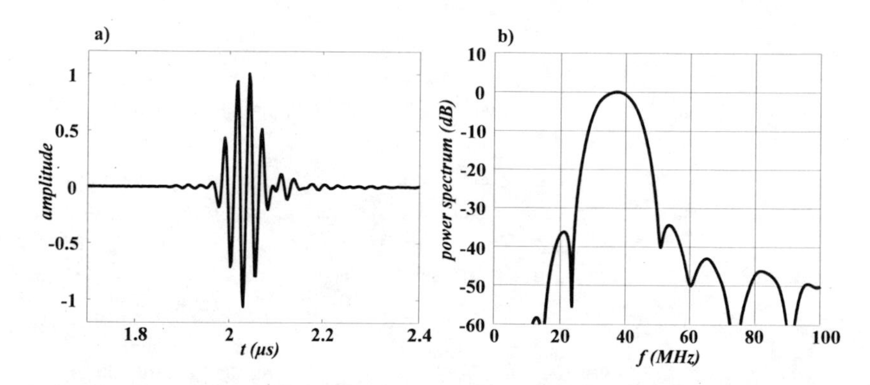

Figure 5.3: Echo from an acrylic plate acquired with a 40 MHz transducer. a): Pulse wave form. b): Logarithmic power spectrum.

Note that the observed center frequencies are lower than the nominal center frequencies in both cases. The transducer specifications provided by the manufacturer state center frequencies of 26.0-28.9 MHz and 34.7-38.6 MHz, respectively. The measured values are within these frequency ranges.

The values measured for axial resolution are lower than those reported by other groups. In the literature the axial resolution of a 40 MHz transducer is given as 80 µm [165]. This value deviates from the measurements presented here, however, the authors did not describe in detail how the measurements were performed. Values found in the literature for 30 MHz transducers deviate even more, they are in the range from 80 µm [64] to 150 µm [127]. These discrepancies are probably caused by the absence of a standardized measurement protocol for resolution. Some groups measure the resolution with multi-wire phantoms and quantify the resolution by visual inspection of B-mode images [49, 50], which will yield poorer resolution than the FWHM method.

5.2.2 Lateral resolution

The lateral resolution of an ultrasound transducer is determined by the lateral beam width. In order to determine lateral resolution, in this work experiments were performed with a thin polyester filament as a reflector. The diameter of the filament was approximately 12 μm, which is well beyond the wavelength at 40 MHz in water. The filament was placed perpendicular to the beam direction and parallel to the elevational direction. Echoes were acquired with the filament positioned at 1.9 mm from the transducer. This distance was assumed to be beyond the near field range (see Equation 2.4.5) with the following reasoning:

The equation for the near field range can be rewritten with the speed of sound c and the center frequency f_c:

$$N = \frac{D^2}{4 \cdot c} f_c \qquad (5.2.1)$$

With the assumption of $c = 1500\,\mathrm{m/s}$ in water, a transducer diameter of 0.5 mm [64] and the center frequencies in Table 5.1, the near field ranges are 1.3 mm and 1.8 mm, respectively.

The measurements were averaged over five acquisitions. As a measure for the lateral resolution δ_{lat}, the lateral width of the echoes was determined, where the amplitude of the demodulated echoes dropped to half its maximum. The results are summarized in Table 5.2. The measured resolution is compared to values given in the literature.

	Measured lateral resolution	Lateral resolution (results from literature)
30 MHz transducer	0.2 mm	0.25 mm [64]
40 MHz transducer	0.17 mm	0.16 mm [165]

Table 5.2: Results of measurements with a polyester filament.

5.3 Data acquisition setup

Commercially available intravascular ultrasound scanners are used for data acquisition, since the developed methods are to be used in clinical trials. These systems (Clearview Ultra and Galaxy I, both manufactured by Boston Scientific Corp., USA) are equipped with an rf-signal output. The scanners continuously provide analog rf signals (256 A-lines per frame, 30 frames per second). However, no trigger signal for individual A-lines is available. Such a signal is necessary for controlling the analog to digital (A/D) converter used for the experiments (Compuscope 14100, Gage Applied Inc., Canada). Therefore, additional hardware is required to generate triggers for each of the 256 A-lines per frame. In addition, the signals have to be amplified to use the full dynamic range of the A/D converter. Figure 5.4 outlines the hardware setup that was developed and implemented in the context of this work. The A-lines are simultaneously fed to a voltage controlled amplifier (VCA) and a trigger generation unit. The VCA is controlled by a signal generator which creates a signal ramp. This unit operates as a time gain compensation unit (TGC) that compensates depth dependent attenuation of the ultrasound signals. The amplified signals are then band pass filtered, digitized at a sampling rate of 100 MHz and stored on a personal computer (PC). Two different custom made band pass filters were constructed for the 30 MHz and 40 MHz transducers. The trigger generation unit provides trigger signals for each A-line and for each image frame. Each A-line starts with a characteristic ring-down signal, with an amplitude that is significantly higher than the echo signal amplitude. The first slope of each ring-down signal is detected with a Schmitt Trigger circuit and a trigger signal is generated to determine the start of a new A-line. A trigger for the start of an image frame is generated by counting the A-lines with an 8 bit counter.

For continuous data acquisition a versatile trigger interface was developed, comprising a microcontroller [125]. This interface is designed for real-time applications, because it synchronizes the two trigger-signals to a single one for the A/D converter and operates independently from the PC, which is only used to control the unit. The interface allows ECG or pressure gated acquisition and can skip A-lines or complete frames in order to save PC memory. The A/D converter acquires a certain number of samples for a preset number of trigger events before transferring the data to the PC memory over the PCI-bus. Figure 5.5 gives a detailed view of the trigger interface.

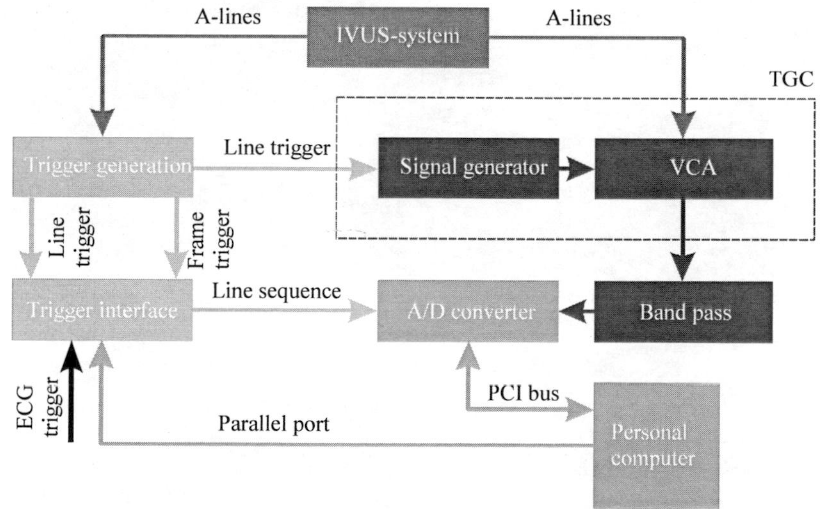

Figure 5.4: Data acquisition setup comprising the IVUS system, signal amplification, a trigger unit and a PC with an A/D converter.

The main function of this unit is to provide a Line sequence trigger for the A/D converter depending on the input trigger signals and user defined presets. At each Line trigger event a certain number of samples are acquired. The output signal must not be delayed by the microcontroller calculations, or a significant delay and jitter would occur in the A/D conversion from line to line. Therefore, the input line trigger is bypassed and directly fed to an AND gate. The gates only have a minimal gate time delay in the order of nanoseconds. Thus the output line sequence will follow the line trigger signal with a negligible constant time delay if the Frame-enable and Line-enable inputs have a logic 1. These two inputs are used to control data acquisition with the microcontroller. Using the parallel port, the controller program can be initialized, modified and reset at any time during data acquisition by the PC. This is an important feature for continuous operation, because acquisition can be suspended during data transfer from the A/D converter to PC memory and can be resumed at the start of the next available frame. This ensures that only a minimum number of frames are dropped during data transfer. The microcontroller is equipped with counters for the Line and Frame signals. The number of A-lines and frames that are acquired and the repetition rate of a sequence can be adjusted freely. Whenever an A-line has to be acquired, the Line enable signal is set to a logic 1, otherwise it is set to 0 and no Line sequence trigger is generated. The Frame trigger is latched in order to keep a logic 1 for the duration of a frame.

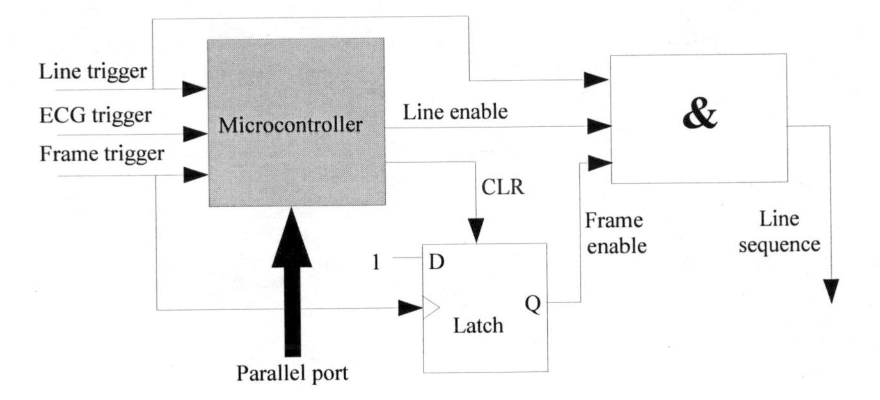

Figure 5.5: Trigger interface comprising a microcontroller (Microchip PIC 16C55), a latch and a three input AND gate.

The timing diagram in Figure 5.6 illustrates this behavior with an example. The Line trigger continuously changes states. The microcontroller is preset to skip the first A-line and then acquire every other line. The controller sets the Line enable signal to a logic 1 only after a Frame trigger was recorded and the first Line trigger has passed. It then changes states as depicted, which results in the desired Line sequence. Note that the Line sequence never starts before a Frame trigger was recorded. This ensures that frames are always aligned with each other, even if the acquisition was suspended for data transfer to PC memory. The sequence of frames can be controlled by the clear input (CLR) of the latch. If a complete frame is to be skipped, CLR is simply set to a logic 0 and the line sequence signal is bound to a logic 0.

Custom software was developed for signal processing and to control the data acquisition [125, 143]. Image frames can be acquired either continuously or as a block of data. In continuous mode two or more consecutive frames are acquired and transferred to the PC memory for further processing. After the data transfer a strain image is calculated and displayed on the screen. Since the data acquisition operates independently of the PC, the next image sequence can be acquired simultaneously. The setup can process and display up to 7 strain images per second in real-time. In the block mode a number of consecutive frames is acquired and stored in the A/D converter onboard memory. The data transfer is initiated after the desired number of frames was stored. This mode only allows data post-processing. This mode of operation is useful for off-line strain image calculation.

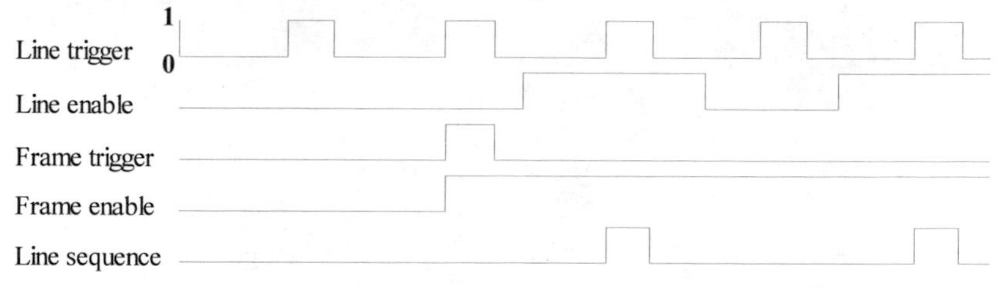

Figure 5.6: Example of a timing diagram (signal duty cycles are not to scale)

5.4 Non-uniform rotational distortion (NURD)

The single element transducers are mounted on a drive shaft which continuously rotates in a catheter sheath during image acquisition, driven by an external motor. The catheter has to be long enough to reach the coronary vessel system. At the same time it has to be flexible, because the vessels are tortuous. Due to its length and flexibility the drive shaft is not torsionally rigid. Thus, friction between drive shaft and the outer tube leads to variations in angular rotation velocity. When displaying the ultrasound images, a constant angular velocity is assumed. Velocity variations lead to image distortions, because the image is either stretched or compressed in angular direction. This effect can be observed in Figure 5.7. At eleven and one o'clock the image is stretched, which is presumably caused by a decrease of the rotation speed in that sector.

These distortions have been quantified experimentally by Ten Hoff et al. [191]. They developed an experimental setup for simultaneous measurement of motor and catheter tip rotation speed. It was shown that an angular error occurs, which can be divided into three components. A constant offset, periodic velocity variations and a stochastic velocity error component. The constant offset does not cause image distortion, while the other two components lead to local image compression or expansion in angular direction. It was also shown that the errors are reduced with increased rotation speed. However, at high rotation speeds echoes at larger depths might not be received accurately since the ultrasound beam is rotated significantly between pulse transmission and receive. This imposes an upper limit on rotation speeds. Another source of errors is the catheter angulation that occurs during in vivo imaging. The arterial system is tortuous and the shaft is bent significantly at various locations. In several phantom studies it was shown that angle distortions increase with progressive catheter angulation [89, 91, 191]. It was shown that especially the periodic error increased with bent catheters, while the stochastic error was reported to decrease [191].

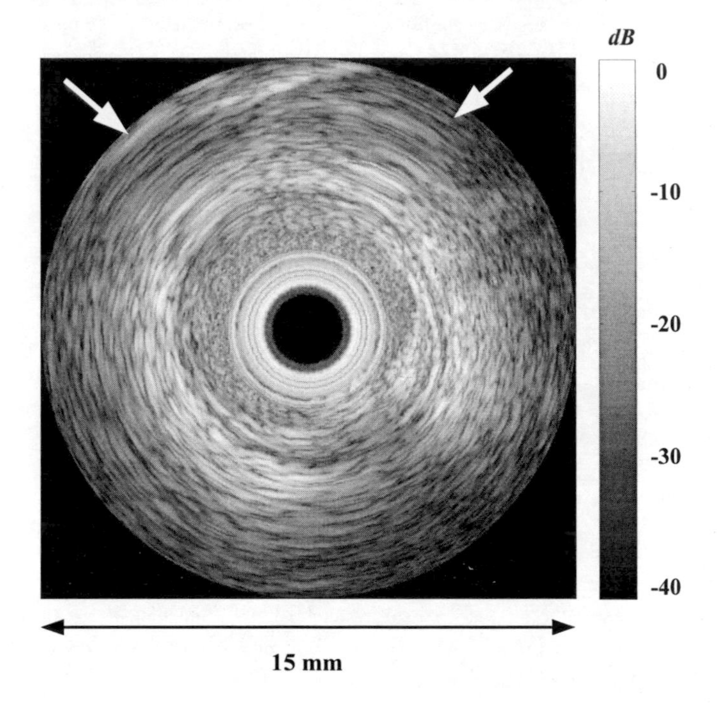

Figure 5.7: IVUS image of a coronary artery acquired in vivo with a rotating transducer. NURD artifacts are visible at 11 and 1 o'clock.

In conjunction with strain imaging NURD artifacts may pose a severe limitation. The method heavily depends on sufficiently high image correlation and is very sensitive to undesired motion. In many cases distortions are hardly visible in the B-mode images, but strain estimations are still erroneous due to decorrelation. The constant offset and periodic velocity variations in phase with the frame rate do not have a significant impact on the correlation of consecutive images, since the frame to frame variation is minimal and images are equally distorted. Velocity variations out of phase with the frame rate and the stochastic error that varies from frame to frame will degrade strain imaging and cause decorrelation because the ultrasound beams of consecutive frames are not aligned. This effect is drafted in Figure 5.8. The variations in angular speed cause a misalignment of beams by an angle φ. The beams only overlap in a certain region.

In these cases decorrelation is caused by two effects: First, the misalignment causes displacements in angular direction, i.e. the image is rotated in the corresponding sector. Second, if this displacement is not an integer multiple of the A-line spacing, the tissue is insonified at a different angle. This causes a change in speckle patterns [83, 128], which reduces correlation. The first effect can be compensated by beam realignment with block matching algorithms, which will be presented later in this chapter. The second is a physical limitation and cannot be compensated.

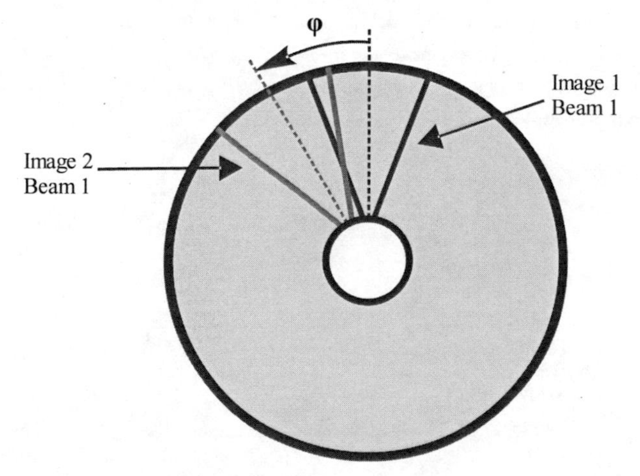

Figure 5.8: Misalignment of beams of consecutive images due to non-uniform rotation. Decorrelation occurs due to this effect.

5.4.1 Influence of catheter angulation on NURD

5.4.1.1 Methods

In order to assess the influence of NURD on image correlation, phantom experiments have been performed. In this work, five imaging catheters equipped with transducers of 40 MHz center frequency were analyzed. Two of the imaging catheters were unused, while the remaining three have been used previously in a clinical exam. For the experiments each imaging catheter was placed in a water tank, with the distal tip at least 20 cm away from the tank's insertion sheath to allow free movement of the transducer. A homogeneous cylindrical phantom (3 mm inner diameter, 6 cm length) was placed in the tank without constriction. The phantom was made from polyvinyl alcohol cryogel (PVA), the properties of vascular PVA phantoms are described in [66]. In order to assess the influence of catheter angulation, the experiments were performed with three guiding catheters of different angularity. The guiding catheters (Figure 5.9) are commercially available and used in clinical routine. They represent typical bends that can occur during in vivo experiments. The transducer tip was placed inside the phantom without constrictions. The data were acquired without intraluminal pressure variations. The data acquisition was performed at least two minutes after catheter placement to minimize the effect of water motion in the tank. Thus signal decorrelation could only result from system noise or irregular transducer movement due to NURD.

Ten consecutive images were recorded for each transducer position. The transducer was pulled back within the imaging catheter sheath by steps of 1 cm and the acquisition was repeated four times. This was done to investigate if NURD depends on specific transducer positions within the sheath. Prior to each acquisition the transducer sheath was flushed with water to ensure that no artifacts from air bubbles within the sheath are present. For each combination of imaging catheter and guiding catheter the acquisition procedure was repeated, resulting in a total number of $3 \cdot 5 \cdot 4 \cdot 10 = 600$ data sets.

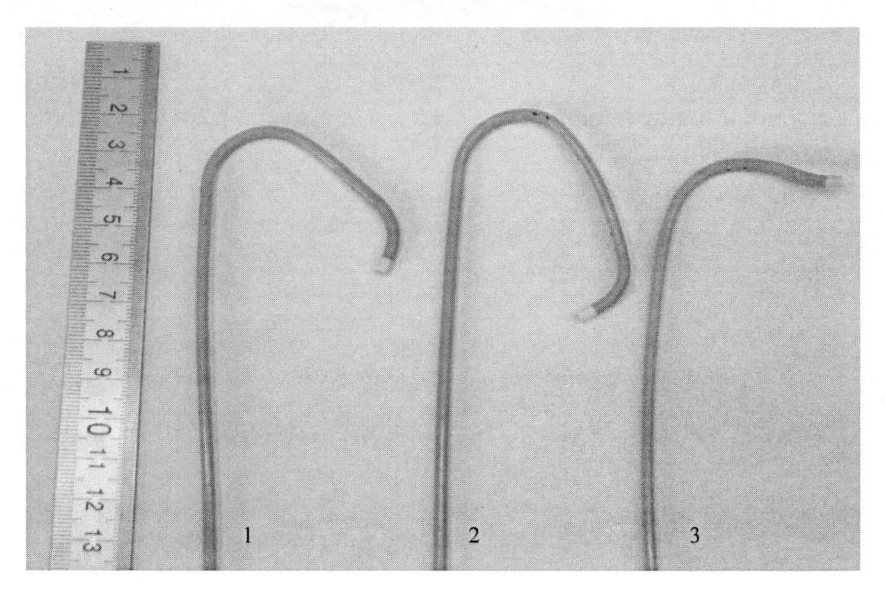

Figure 5.9: Guiding catheters used in this study

Figure 5.10 exemplarily shows one B-mode image of a phantom. The catheter was located in the lumen in an eccentric position. The dark areas inside and outside the phantom are regions of water. The bright area at the top of the image is a signal ring-down artifact, caused by transducer ringing and multiple reflections at the catheter shaft. The data acquired in this work exhibited an extended artifact that was caused by saturation of the amplifier in the experimental setup. This artifact sometimes covered parts of the tissue. Throughout this work care was taken that data segments covered by the artifact were not used for analysis. In the example in Figure 5.10, only data within the white box were considered for further processing.

The artifacts were assessed by evaluating the local normalized cross correlation function of frame pairs from an image sequence. All combinations of frame pairs were analyzed in each data set of 10 frames. The number of combinations can be calculated by the binomial coefficient [17]:

$$\binom{n}{k} = \frac{n!}{(n-k)! \cdot k!} \tag{5.4.1}$$

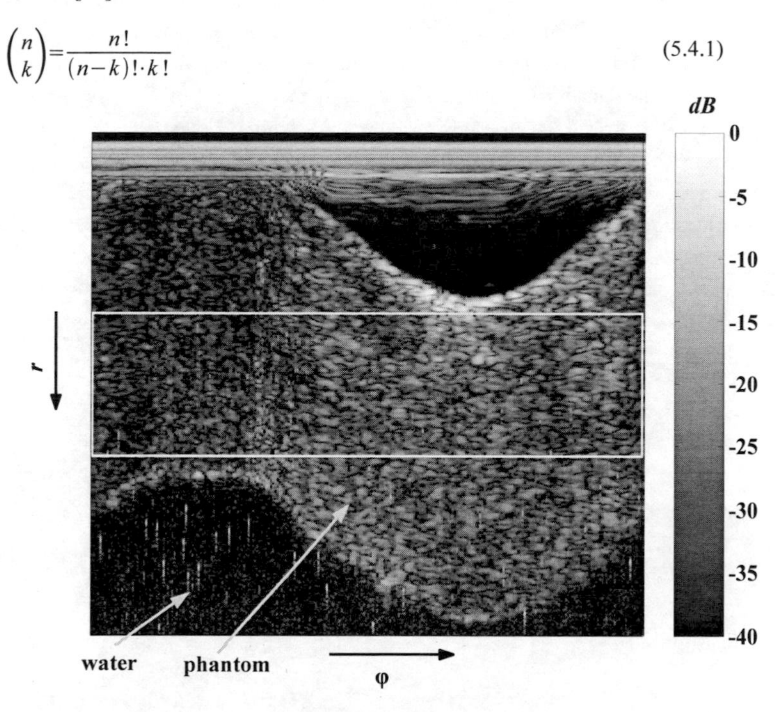

Figure 5.10: B-mode image of a PVA phantom in polar coordinates. The white box indicates the area that was used for data analysis.

The binomial coefficient gives the number of *k*-subsets out of a set of *n* distinct elements. For $n=10$ and $k=2$ Equation (5.4.1) yields 45 combinations.

For cross correlation analysis, consider $x_{1b}(k, \varphi_j)$ and $x_{2b}(k, \varphi_j)$ to be a pair of A-lines from consecutive frames in baseband representation. Here, φ_j denotes the jth angular position $(j=1..256)$. A measure of similarity in a time window centered around k_i is given by the absolute value of the normalized cross correlation function at zero lag, which is calculated as:

$$r_{norm}(k_i,\varphi_j)=\frac{\left|\sum_{l=k_i-M/2}^{k_i+M/2-1} x_{1b}^{*}(l+\tau_{k_i},\varphi_j)\cdot x_{2b}(l,\varphi_j)\right|}{\sqrt{\sum_{l=k_i-M/2}^{k_i+M/2-1}(x_{1b}(l+\tau_{k_i},\varphi_j))^2\cdot\sum_{l=k_i-M/2}^{k_i+M/2-1}(x_{2b}(l,\varphi_j))^2}} \quad (5.4.2)$$

Due to the normalization r_{norm} equals 1 if the signals are identical. Since this study focuses on decorrelation due to lateral motion only, axial time shifts within the windows caused by catheter motion or digitization jitter were corrected to ensure maximum correlation. For this task, the radial shift τ_{k_i} of the signals was estimated in each signal window according to Equation (3.3.13). In Equation (5.4.2) the signal x_{1b} is then shifted by τ_{k_i} for compensation. This equation was evaluated in consecutive windows of length M along the radial direction. In this application a window size of 7 wavelengths was chosen with 75% window overlap, these values were determined empirically. Thus, an image with a local distribution of r_{norm} is formed as exemplarily shown in Figure 5.11. A stripe pattern with radial bands of reduced correlation is visible in this image. In order to assess the decorrelation due to NURD, for each frame pair the percentage of values lower than a threshold $r_{norm}<0.9$ was determined.

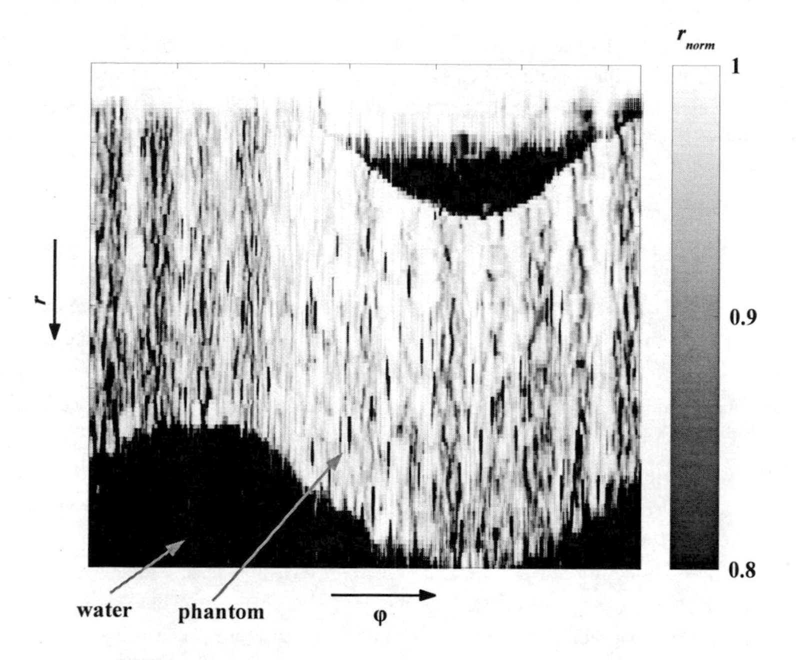

Figure 5.11: Distribution of r_{norm} calculated from consecutive frames according to Equation (5.4.2). Bands of reduced correlation are visible throughout the phantom area.

5.4.1.2 Results and discussion

The following diagrams show the results for different combinations of imaging catheter and guiding catheter. The imaging catheters number one and two were unused, while the others have been used once before. The influence of catheter angulation for each imaging catheter is displayed in Figure 5.12. The abscissa of each diagram shows the guiding catheter number according to Figure 5.9, the ordinate displays the mean and standard deviation of the percentage of r_{norm} values with $r_{norm}<0.9$. In Figure 5.13 the same results are presented, but this time in a separate diagram for each guiding catheter. Here, the percentage of $r_{norm}<0.9$ is plotted versus the imaging catheter number. In all cases the results show that less than 25% of the values were below the threshold. Figure 5.14 exemplarily shows the measurement results for an imaging/guiding catheter combination. The percentage of values below the threshold is given for all frame pairs of a data set, each plot represents a specific transducer position within the imaging catheter sheath. The dashed line represents a transducer position where in all frame pairs more than 15% of the r_{norm} values were below the threshold.

It is expected that progressive catheter angulation leads to increased NURD and thus to decorrelation. However, the results in Figure 5.12 show no clear relationship between catheter angulation and reduced correlation. The plots for imaging catheter one and four show that with guiding catheter two decorrelation is slightly reduced. However, this is the guiding catheter with the smallest bend radius. The guiding catheters used in this study represent realistic bends, but the results suggest that the radii were not small enough to cause significant correlation changes due to NURD. This is in accordance with the results of a study performed by Kearney et al. [89], where no significant relationship between NURD and catheter angulation was found.

The plots in Figure 5.13 suggest that the results are more dependent on individual imaging catheter properties. Imaging catheter three shows significant decorrelation in combination with guiding catheters one and two. For imaging catheter one, an average of more than 5% of the values are below the threshold in combination with guiding catheters one and three. The standard deviation is wide in those cases. Interestingly, imaging catheter one was previously unused but shows increased decorrelation in several cases. Thus, the performance cannot be related to age or prior use, but rather to manufacturing variations.

The plots in Figure 5.14 illustrate that correlation varies with transducer position and from frame to frame. The dashed line in the diagram represents a specific transducer position and shows higher values than the three other graphs. This can be explained by friction that varies when pulling back the transducer within the sheath. It does not cause a fundamental problem for correlation based strain imaging since the catheter can be repositioned during clinical examination. The diagram also shows frame to frame variations. Within a sequence of ten images the values vary by more than 15%. This can only be related to NURD that varies over time, since no external motion was present that could cause decorrelation. This effect poses a severe limitation for correlation analysis, since it cannot be avoided through user interaction.

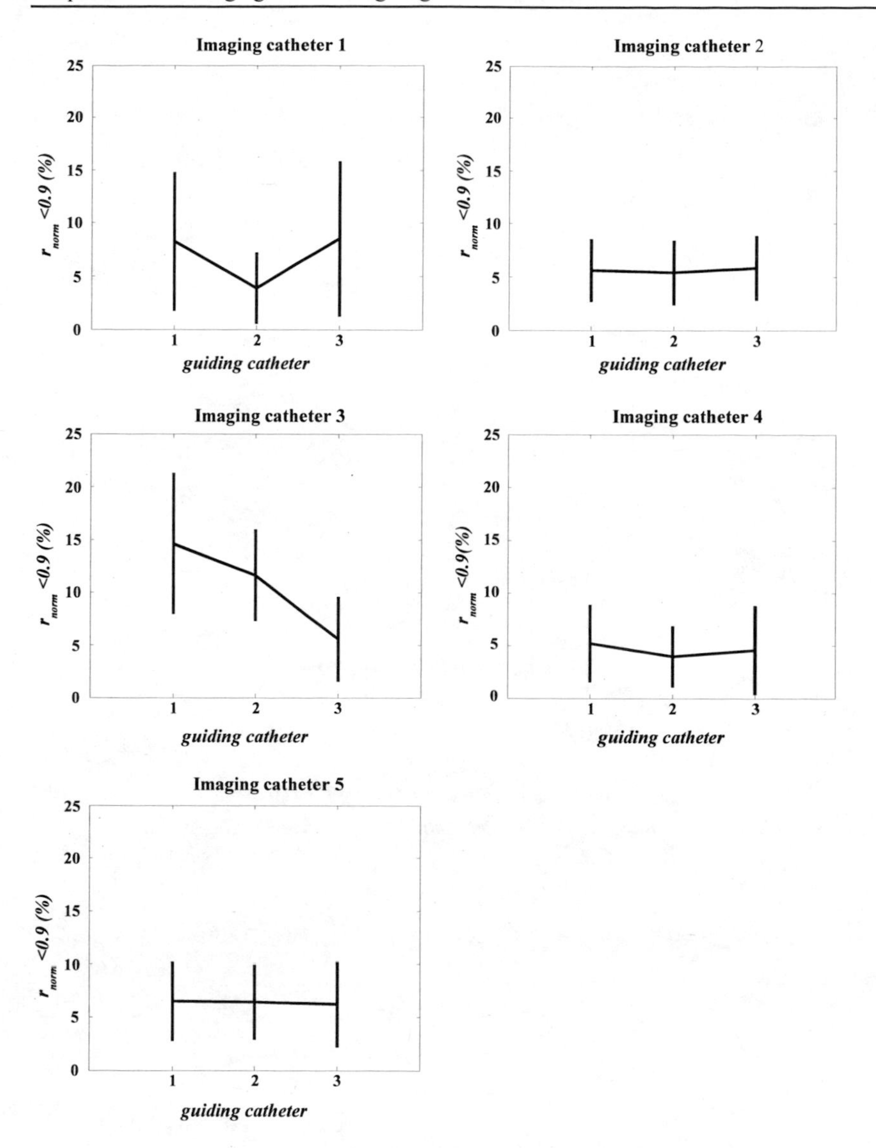

Figure 5.12: Mean and standard deviation of the percentage of segments with $r_{norm}<0.9$ *displayed for each imaging catheter in combination with the three guiding catheters.*

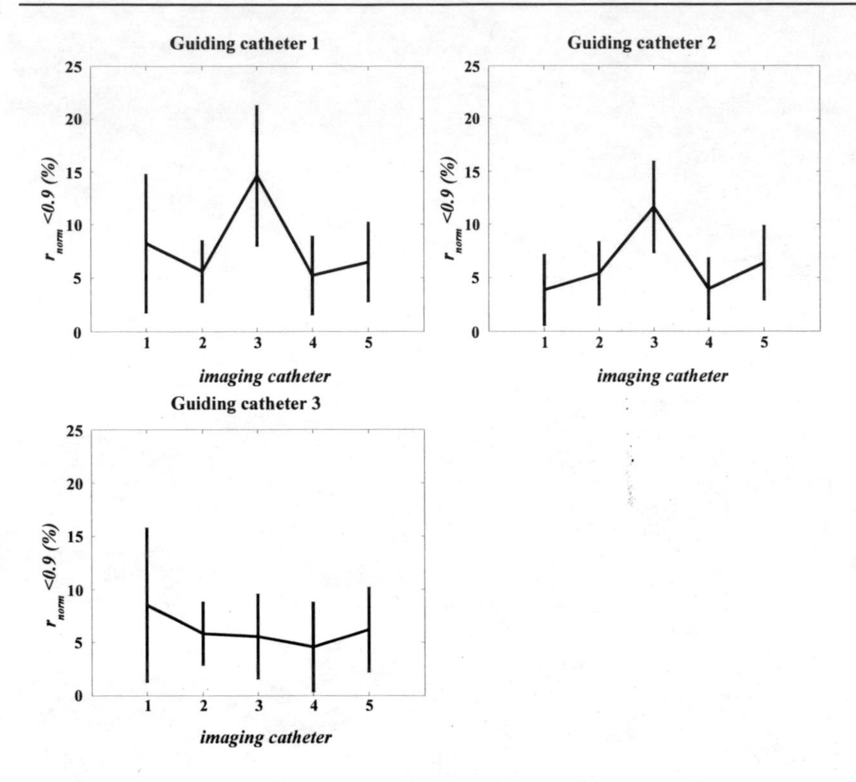

Figure 5.13: Mean and standard deviation of the percentage of segments with $r_{norm}<0.9$ *displayed for each guiding catheter in combination with the five imaging catheters.*

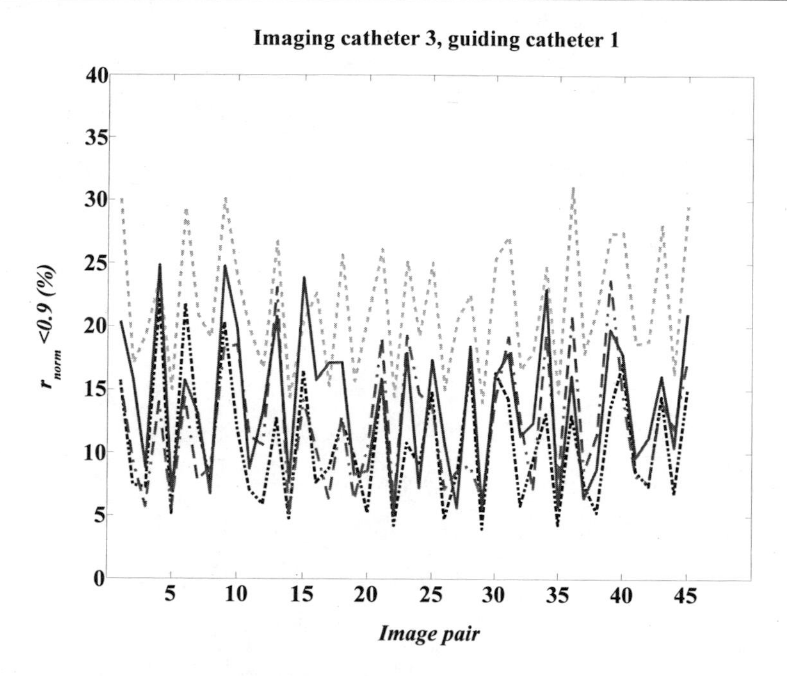

Figure 5.14: Results for the combination of imaging catheter three with guiding catheter one. The percentage of segments with $r_{norm}<0.9$ *is plotted for all combinations of frame pairs. Each graph represents a different transducer position within the imaging catheter sheath.*

5.4.2 Dependence of artifacts on the motor drive

Variations in rotation speed are not only dependent on the mechanical characteristics of the imaging catheter, but also on the quality of the motor drive. In contrast to the imaging catheters, the motor drive is not a disposable product and can be worn out by multiple use. Since the ultrasound system is classified as a medical grade system, no custom made motors optimized for uniform rotation can be used in clinical examinations. In order to demonstrate the influence of different motor drives on image correlation, a phantom experiment was performed with two motors. As described in the previous section, the acquisitions were performed in a water tank with a PVA phantom. A 30 MHz imaging catheter was placed in the phantom lumen without constriction, in combination with guiding catheter three. First, a motor that was in laboratory use for three months was connected and ten consecutive images were acquired. Next, a previously unused motor was connected, taking care that the position of the imaging catheter in the water tank remained unchanged. A second set of ten images was acquired with this motor. The data were analyzed as described in the previous section, except that a threshold of 0.95 was applied for r_{norm} because the overall correlation was higher with this particular imaging catheter. For each set of ten images all combinations of image pairs were evaluated, resulting in 45 correlation images. The results are plotted in Figure 5.15 for both cases. The solid plot shows the results for data acquired with the unused motor, results for the used motor are represented by the dashed plot. Mean and standard deviation of the percentage of values below the threshold are summarized in Table 5.3.

This example clearly shows that the mechanical rotation performance of the motor drive has an impact on image correlation. Although the overall correlation is higher than in the study of the previous section, the differences of the two motors are substantial. The consequence for clinical trials is that motor performance has to be verified periodically.

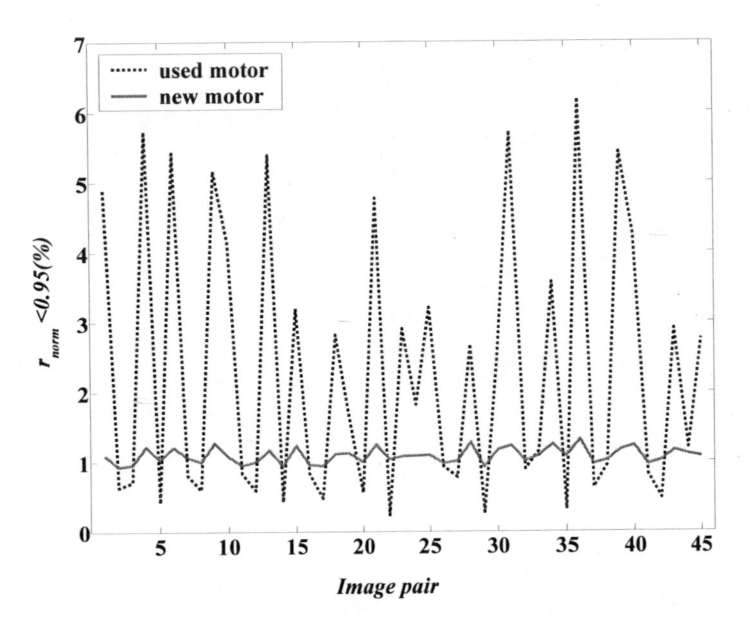

Figure 5.15: Evaluation of data acquired with two different motor drives. The graphs show the percentage of segments with $r_{norm}<0.95$ *plotted for 45 combinations of frame pairs.*

$r_{norm}<0.95$	μ(%)	σ(%)
Used motor	2.28	1.93
New motor	1.09	0.11

Table 5.3: Mean and standard deviation of the percentage of $r_{norm}<0.95$.

5.4.3 Correction of NURD artifacts

IVUS strain imaging heavily depends on sufficiently high image correlation. The correlation of consecutive IVUS images can be improved by realignment of beams. In previous studies beam realignment was investigated with array transducers [82]. However, no results were reported on rotating single element transducers which are prone to NURD. In this section, the effect of beam realignment on image correlation is assessed experimentally, initial experiments have been reported in [147].

5.4.3.1 Methods

Using the acquisition scheme and data described in chapter 5.4.1, the shift of beams in lateral direction is estimated and corrected by beam realignment. The beam shift is estimated from envelope detected data with a Sum of Absolute Difference (SAD) algorithm. In many cases the estimated lateral shift did not exceed one beam. The data were therefore interpolated in lateral direction in order to assess sub-beam shift. Linear interpolation was applied, the rf A-lines were interpolated in lateral direction by a factor of five to provide sufficient sub-beam resolution. After that, the rf signals were converted into baseband signals according to Equation (3.3.9). Data analysis was performed in one dimensional windows sliding across the beams. Prior to the lateral shift estimation, the axial shift of the signal pairs in each window was compensated as described in the previous section (shift τ_{k_i} in Equation 5.4.2). Again, this was done to minimize errors introduced by axial shift, since only decorrelation due to angle mismatch was investigated. In order to obtain envelope detected (demodulated) data, the absolute value of the base band signals was calculated. Lateral displacement was estimated by calculating the SAD in one dimensional windows of size M' sliding across signals in radial direction. The window size was set to $M'=256$ samples, the overlap was 80%. These values were determined empirically with focus on sufficient correlation. Values in each data window were compared to the neighboring windows from the following frame. The minimum SAD value indicated the best match and thus the lateral shift:

$$SAD_{min}(k_i, j) = \min_{v} \left[\sum_{m=0}^{M'-1} \left| x_{1D}(k_i+m, j) - x_{2D}(k_i+m, j+v) \right| \right] \qquad (5.4.3)$$

In this equation, x_{1D} and x_{2D} denote a pair of demodulated A-lines from two consecutive interpolated frames. The value k_i represents the radial window position, j denotes the A-line index and v was varied in the interval [-6, 6] for a lateral search of the minimum. For each window position the lateral displacement $v_{min}(k_i, j)$ of the best matching pair was recorded. Finally, a global lateral shift for each A-line was determined by averaging the displacement values along a line. Thus, for each line a global displacement value was found. The A-lines were then realigned according to the calculated displacement. For the analysis of the effects of beam realignment, the same evaluation procedure as in the previous section was applied and r_{norm} was calculated according to Equation (5.4.2) before and after correction. Since the beam realignment procedure was computationally expensive, only consecutive frames were evaluated instead of calculating all permutations as described by Equation (5.4.1). Thus, nine frame pairs were evaluated for each series of ten frames.

5.4.3.2 Results and discussion

The results demonstrate that lateral shift can be corrected by beam realignment, which improves image correlation. Figure 5.16 exemplarily shows results obtained from one frame pair. Images of the local distribution of r_{norm} before and after beam realignment are displayed side by side. The diagram a) shows the uncorrected case with radial bands of reduced correlation. After beam realignment the correlation is increased and appears more uniform within the phantom, as can be seen in diagram b). The Figures 5.17 and 5.18 show the correlation results for all combinations of guiding catheters and imaging catheters. As in the previous section, the results are catheter dependent. For all combinations, mean values and standard deviations of $r_{norm} < 0.9$ are reduced by realignment, which demonstrates that correlation is improved.

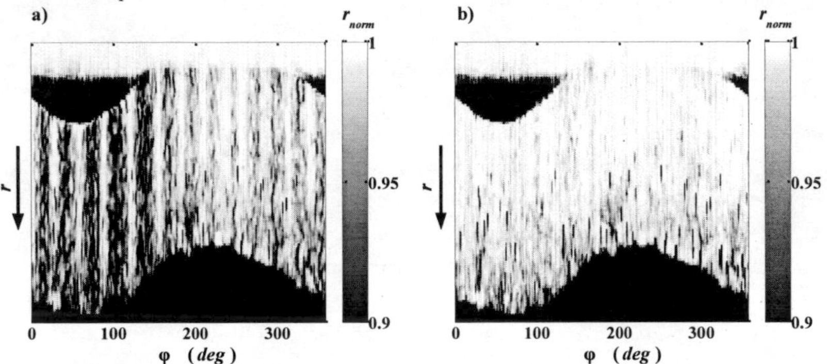

Figure 5.16:Distribution of r_{norm} calculated from consecutive frames according to Equation 5.4.2. a): No lateral correction was applied, bands of reduced correlation are visible throughout the phantom area. b): Lateral correction was applied by realignment of beams.

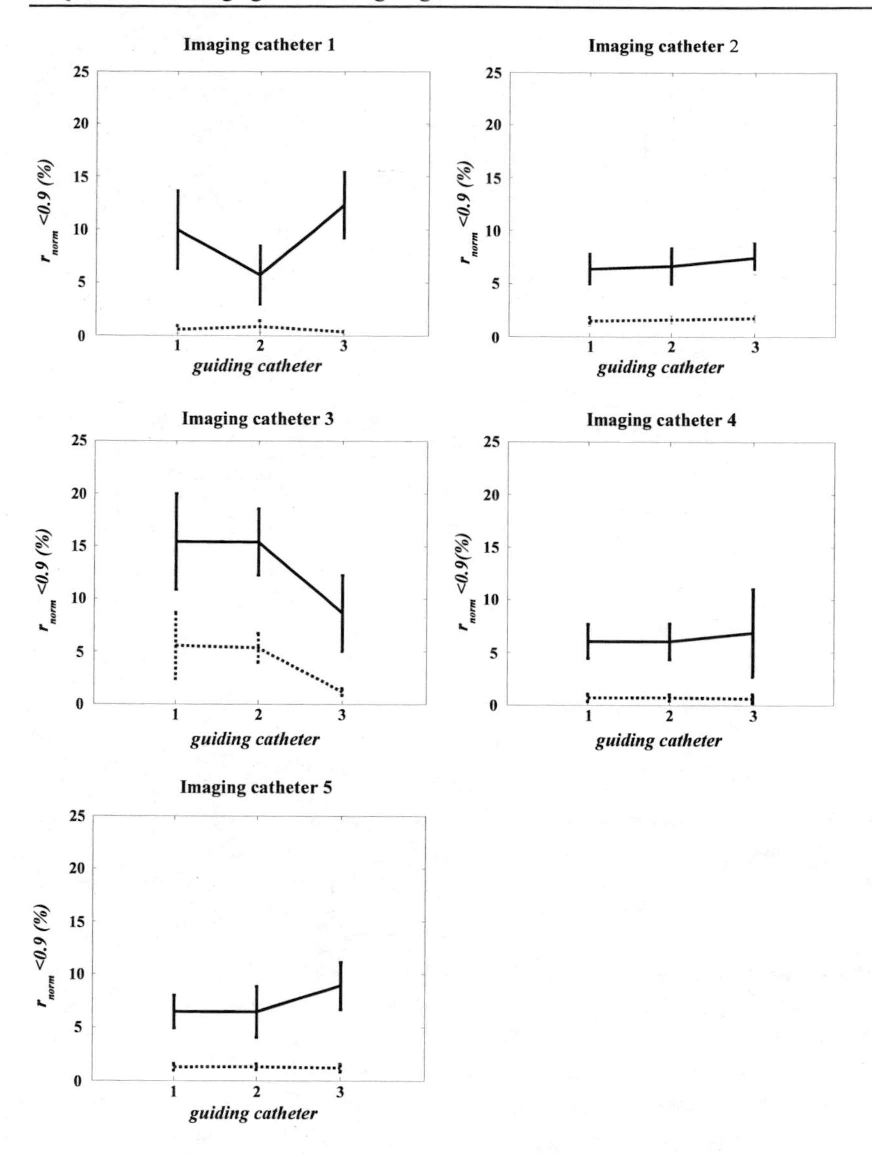

Figure 5.17: Mean and standard deviation of the percentage of segments with r_{norm}<0.9 *displayed for each imaging catheter in combination with the three guiding catheters. The solid lines represent results without lateral correction, the dashed lines show results of corrected data.*

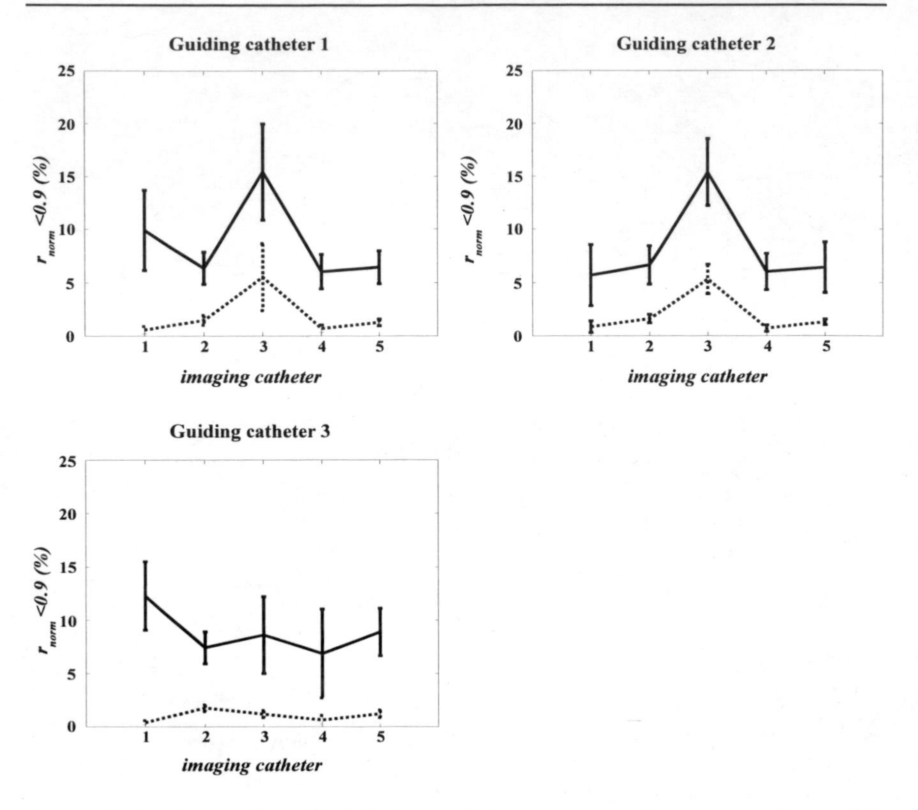

Figure 5.18: Mean and standard deviation of the percentage of segments with r_{norm}<0.9 *displayed for each guiding catheter in combination with the five imaging catheters. The solid lines represent results without lateral correction, the dashed lines show results of corrected data.*

The estimated lateral beam shift was within the limits of ± 1 beams. Figure 5.19 exemplarily shows a plot of the estimated shift versus the angle of rotation. The left diagram displays the lateral shift estimation over the angle obtained from one pair of consecutive frames. The right diagram shows the shift estimates of consecutive frames in concatenation (frames 1-2, 2-3, ... 9-10). The shift varies over the angle. Besides a noise component, the shift also has a component that changes direction in a periodic manner, as can be seen in the left diagram of Figure 5.19. The analysis of image sequences reveals that the periodic pattern is present in all acquired image pairs, regardless of the transducer in use. The cycle duration of the periodic shift does not change with different transducers, the analysis of all frame pairs yields 6.3 ± 0.18 cycles per frame. A possible explanation for this observation is that the rotation velocity changes periodically, but not with the same frequency as the frame rate. Thus, from frame to frame the phase of the rotation speed variation is different at a given location and causes beam misalignment. This effect may be ascribed to motor imperfections, since it is independent of the catheter in use. Also, if this effect was caused solely by catheter friction, the shift is expected to be highly irregular. The right diagram in Figure 5.19 suggests that an additional low frequency modulation is present in a series of consecutive frames. This effect may be ascribed to non-uniform rotation at a frequency lower than the frame rate.

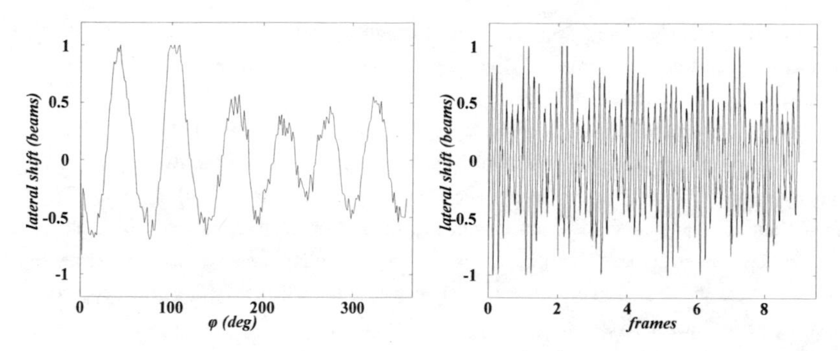

Figure 5.19: Estimated mean lateral shift. Left: Shift of the beams plotted versus the beam angle for one pair of consecutive frames. Right: Concatenation of shift estimates for nine consecutive frame pairs.

5.4.4 Conclusions

The experimental results show that NURD is a complex phenomenon and depends on several factors. There is no clear indication that NURD increases monotonically with reduced catheter bend angles. However, the mechanical properties of motors and individual catheters have a prominent impact on NURD. Oscillating beam shifts are observed which are possibly related to the motor characteristics. With some catheters image correlation is significantly reduced, which suggests that friction varies with each catheter. Correlation errors can be reduced by beam realignment. The periodic shifts are efficiently corrected by this method, but it does not compensate for equipment specific NURD in all cases. In an in-vivo environment the correction algorithm will suffer from artifacts due to tissue motion. Thus, for strain imaging it is crucial to select equipment that yields an acceptable degree of uniform rotation. In the clinical application, only sterile, disposable catheters can be used. The mechanical transducer characteristics can therefore only be assessed after image acquisition. Data have to be discarded in cases of severe NURD.

5.5 Phantom experiments

In order to evaluate the strain imaging algorithms developed in chapter 3.3, phantom experiments were performed under controlled pressure conditions.

5.5.1 Methods

Vessel mimicking phantoms were created from Polyvinyl Alcohol Cryogel (PVA) as described in chapter 4.3. Cylindric two layer phantoms of different geometries were manufactured. Figure 5.20 displays the cross-sections of phantoms used for strain imaging. A phantom with an eccentric circular inner layer is outlined in diagram a). The eccentricity of the inner layer was introduced to distinguish the strain differences of the two layers from the geometry dependent radial strain decay (see chapter 3.2). The diagram b) shows a phantom with a quadratic inner layer concentric with the lumen center. The diagram c) displays the cylindric phantom structure. The outer layers of both phantoms underwent three freeze-thaw cycles and were stiffer than the inner layers (two freeze-thaw cycles). Since the scope of this work comprises qualitative analysis only, the elastic moduli of the materials were not determined.

The experiments were performed in a water tank. The experimental setup is outlined in Figure 5.21. The phantom was mounted on a holder which was placed in the tank. The holder was connected to a water column. The pressure inside the phantom lumen was varied by changing the height of the water column. The imaging catheter was inserted through a sheath and placed in the phantom lumen, while effort was made to center the catheter within the lumen. The acquisitions were performed under static pressure conditions, i.e. the pressure level was varied in-between acquisitions and data of an image were acquired at a constant pressure level.

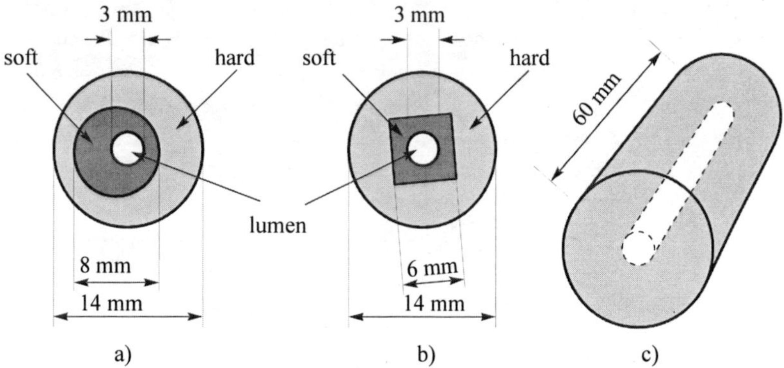

Figure 5.20: Geometry of cylindric two-layer vessel phantoms. a): Circular eccentric soft inner layer. b): Quadratic soft inner layer. c) Cylindric structure.

Data acquisition was performed with the acquisition setup described in chapter 5.3. Single element transducers with 30 MHz as well as 40 MHz center frequencies were used. Care was taken that only catheters yielding a low degree of NURD were used for the phantom study. Catheters with NURD were excluded from the study based on the visual inspection of correlation images. In order to demonstrate the feasibility of the developed 1-D strain estimation algorithm, the calculations were performed without correction for motion in angular direction. The contour detection required for strain estimation was done by applying a threshold to the rf-data. Radial strain was calculated with the algorithms described in chapter 3.3.

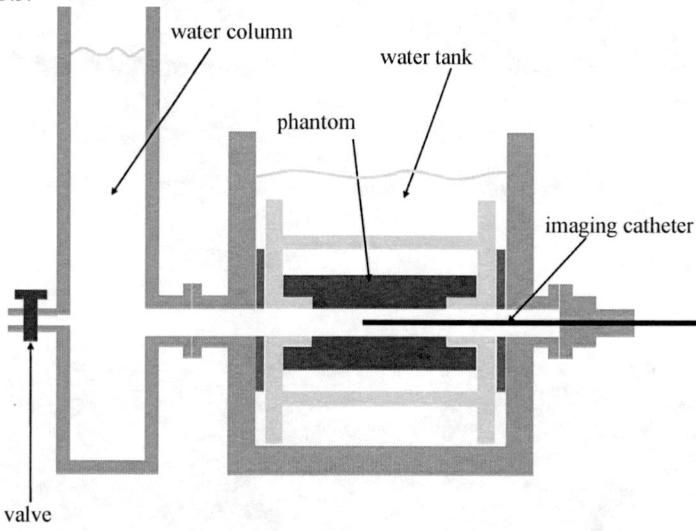

Figure 5.21: Experimental setup. The pressure inside the phantom lumen changes with the height of the water column.

5.5.2 Results and discussion

Figure 5.22 shows the B-mode image of a two layer phantom along with a strain image, obtained with a 30 MHz imaging catheter. The pressure difference between the acquisitions was 0.7 mmHg. The shift of A-line pairs was calculated with a window size of 11 wavelengths, subsequent windows overlapped by 65%. The least squares filter for strain calculation comprised $N_s=15$ displacement samples. A 3x3 median filter was applied to the strain image. The strain is color coded with strain values ranging from 0% to 0.8%. The two layers were constructed with different scatterer concentrations, thus the soft layer is visible as a dark region in the B-mode image. In the strain image, the inner layer can clearly be distinguished from the outer part by a higher strain. The geometry dependent decrease of the strain with the radius is also visible.

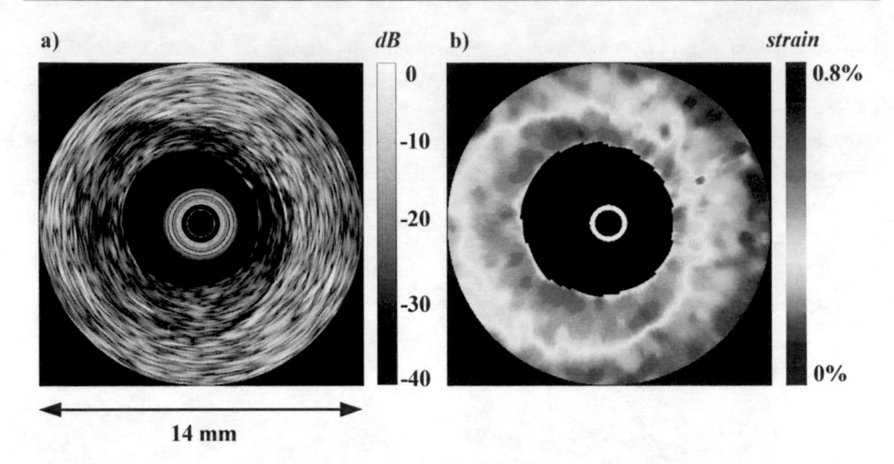

Figure 5.22: B-mode image (a) and corresponding strain image (b) of a two layer PVA phantom (see Figure 5.20 a). The data were acquired with a 30 MHz imaging catheter.

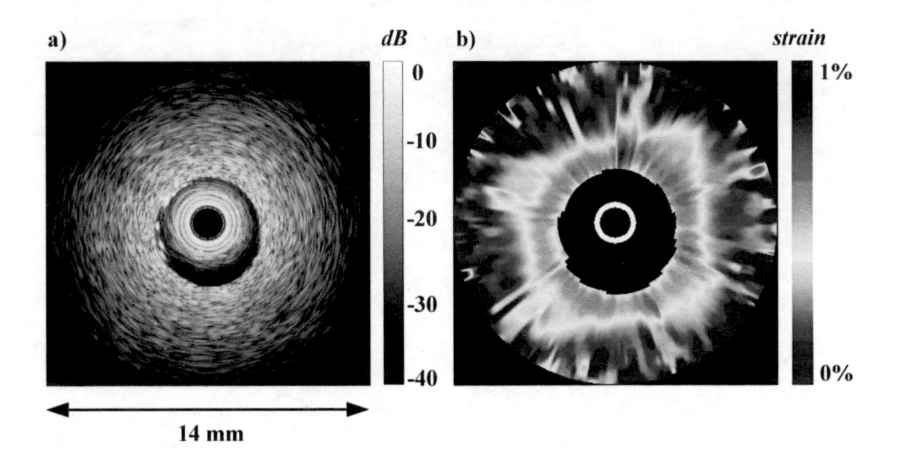

Figure 5.23:B-mode image (a) and corresponding strain image (b) of the two layer PVA phantom (see Figure 5.20 b). The data were acquired with a 40 MHz imaging catheter.

Figure 5.23 displays the B-mode image and the strain image of a phantom with a quadratic soft inner layer. The data were acquired with a 40 MHz imaging catheter. The pressure difference between the acquisitions was 0.8 mmHg. The shift between A-lines was calculated with a window size of 14 wavelengths and 65%. overlap. The filter for strain calculation had a window size of $N_s = 15$ samples. A 3x3 median filter was also applied to this strain image. In this case, both layers contained the same scatterer concentration and thus cannot be distinguished in the B-mode image. The shape of the quadratic inclusion is preserved in the strain image, visible as an area of elevated strain. The quadratic shape is slightly distorted, which results from the applied intraluminal pressure. In both strain images the lumen appears larger than in the B-mode images. This effect is inherent to the differentiator filter used in this approach. Due to the filter ringing, strain directly at the lumen-tissue boundary cannot be calculated. This part of the image was blanked out.

These results show that strain imaging is feasible with the described methods. The differences in tissue stiffness can be qualitatively displayed as strain images. As described in the previous section, the results are highly dependent on the individual catheter and motor properties. These results were obtained with a motor/catheter combination that exhibited low variations in rotation speed. With some catheters severe decorrelation occurred and strain imaging was not successful. The threshold algorithm applied for luminal border segmentation yielded accurate results due to the low echogenicity of water. Its performance is expected to degrade with in vivo data, because the echogenicity of blood is high beyond 30 MHz.

5.5.3 Conclusions

The described setup is suitable for strain imaging, as shown by the qualitative results. Strain images were calculated without compensation for lateral motion, which illustrates that rotating single element transducers can be used for this task in principle. However, artifacts due to mechanical rotation and the transducer specific errors have to be taken into account when analyzing strain images. The results are not reproducible in all cases when exchanging the catheter or introducing different catheter bends. The imaging performance of each catheter has to be verified at least visually prior to data acquisition.

The applied algorithms calculate strain distributions in real-time, currently at a rate of 7 frames per second. This allows direct verification of the strain images, which is an important advantage. The results can often be improved by repositioning the catheter or by changing the pressure levels in order to avoid decorrelation.

5.6 Strain imaging with arteries in vitro

The phantom experiments described in the previous chapter demonstrate that IVUS strain imaging is feasible. However, human arteries have a complex layered structure. The layers contain smooth muscle cells, collagen and elastic fibers. Thus, the vessel tissue is inhomogeneous and anisotropic. In order to investigate the performance of the developed strain imaging algorithms with such a complex material, in vitro experiments were performed with excised human arteries.

5.6.1 Methods

A carotid artery and a left anterior descending coronary artery were obtained at autopsy. The arteries were dissected with surrounding tissue in order to stabilize the vessels. The experiments were performed in a tank filled with saline solution. The vessels were mounted on a holder which was placed in the tank. In the case of the carotid artery, the holder was connected to a water column. The pressure inside the lumen was varied by changing the height of the water column. A carotid artery was chosen for an initial experiment because it has a wide lumen and no side branches. Thus, the pressure loss was minimal throughout the data acquisition. The experiments with the coronary arteries were performed with a closed loop pump that provided a pulsatile flow, simulating coronary perfusion. The side branches were tied with a suture in order to minimize pressure loss. The imaging catheter was inserted through a sheath and placed in the lumen. A centered catheter position could not be achieved in all cases.

The data were aquired with the acquisition setup described in chapter 5.3. Single element transducers with 30 MHz as well as 40 MHz center frequencies were used (Ultra Cross and Atlantis Pro, Boston Scientific, USA). In the experiment with the closed loop pump, consecutive frames were acquired for 3 seconds in order to cover several cycles. Only catheters showing a low degree of NURD were selected for this study. The lumen segmentation required for strain estimation was performed manually. Radial strain was calculated with the algorithms described in chapter 3.3, no correction for lateral motion was applied.

5.6.2 Results and discussion

Figure 5.24 shows the B-mode image and strain image of the carotid artery. The B-mode image is displayed with 40 dB dynamic range. The pressure difference between acquisitions was 7 mmHg. For the strain image, the window size for shift estimation was 11 wavelengths, subsequent windows overlapped by 65%. A 15 tap least squares filter was applied for strain calculation, the strain image was filtered with a 3x3 median filter.

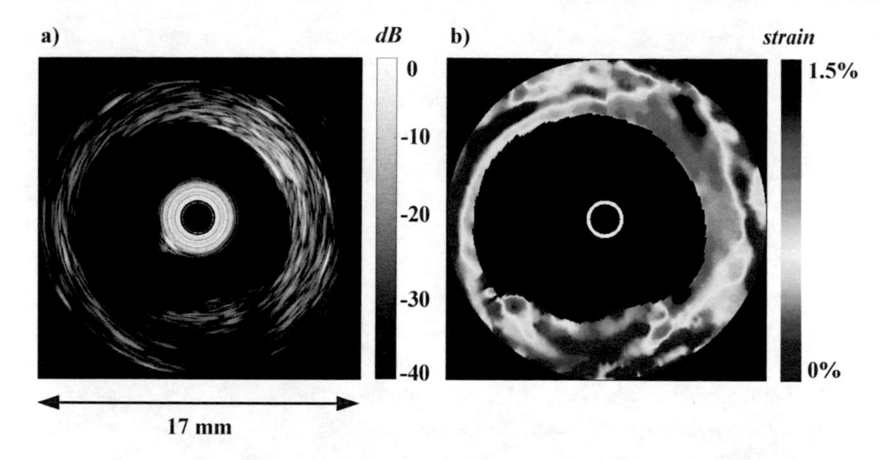

Figure 5.24: B-mode image (a) and corresponding strain image (b) of a carotid artery. The data were acquired with a 30 MHz transducer.

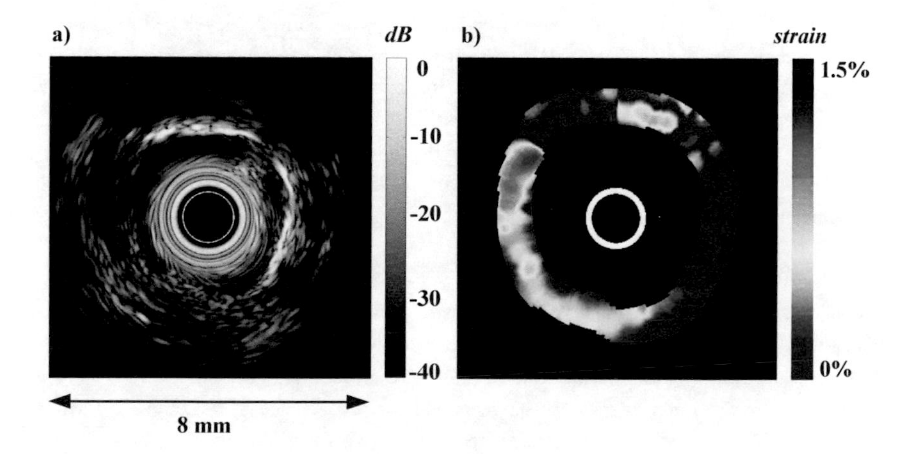

Figure 5.25: B-mode image (a) and corresponding strain image (b) of a coronary artery. The data were acquired with a 40 MHz transducer.

A plaque with an acoustic shadow is visible in the B-mode image between 5 and 7 o'clock. The plaque region can be clearly identified in the strain image as a region of low strain. The high strain region at 2 o'clock presumably corresponds to a layer of loose tissue. The "shoulders" of the plaque exhibit regions of high strain, this effect was also reported by other groups [166, 167].

Figure 5.25 shows images obtained from the coronary artery. The dynamic range of the B-mode image is 40 dB. The window size for shift estimation was 14 wavelengths, the windows overlapped by 65%. The strain was calculated with a 15 tap least squares filter, the image was filtered with a 3x3 median filter. The strain is only displayed in the tissue region close to the transducer, because at deeper radial positions decorrelation occurred due to signal attenuation. Due to the pulsatile flow catheter motion artifacts were introduced. Strain imaging was only successful in those phases of the pulsation cycle where catheter and wall motion was minimal.

The B-mode image in Figure 5.25 exhibits two calcified plaque regions between 11 and 5 o'clock, visible as a bright echo with distal shadows. The two regions are separated around 1 o'clock. The dark area between 9 and 10 o'clock presumably is a dissection. These regions can also be identified in the strain image. The calcified regions exhibit low strain values, because calcifications are harder than the surrounding tissue. The "shoulders" of the plaque are visible as high strain spots. The separation of the two plaque regions around 1 o'clock also exhibits high strain. The dissected tissue appears as an area of high strain around 10 o'clock. Between 5 and 9 o'clock the strain is elevated, in this region the B-mode image exhibits no calcifications.

These results show that in vitro strain imaging is feasible with the developed algorithms. Plaque areas which are visible in the B-mode image and which are presumed to be harder than the surrounding tissue can also be identified in the strain image. They appear as low strain areas. However, the primary goal of intravascular strain imaging is the identification of vulnerable plaques. In the specimens analyzed in this initial study no plaques were found that could be clearly identified as vulnerable. The gold standard for plaque characterization is a histologic analysis, which was not available for these experiments.

5.6.3 Conclusions

The in vitro results suggest that different tissue structures can be characterized by the evaluation of tissue strain. This approach is feasible for human arteries, which have a complex structure. Hard tissue regions such as calcifications can successfully be discriminated from the surrounding tissue. Strain images can be generated in the presence of pulsatile flow, when data acquisitions are performed in cycle phases that exhibit minimal motion artifacts. Further in vitro experiments are required to corroborate these findings. Arteries with vulnerable plaques have to be included in future studies and the results have to be verified by histologic analysis.

5.7 Strain imaging in vivo

The final goal of the described strain imaging algorithms is their application for plaque characterization in vivo. In this section, experiments are presented that were performed in order to investigate strain imaging performance with rotating transducers in vivo. In this case, neither the transducer bend nor the applied pressure difference between acquisitions can be controlled. The heart beat introduces additional in-plane and out-of-plane motion artifacts, during a heart cycle the catheter is shifted back and forth along the vessel axis. The muscle compression also dynamically bends the catheter. Thus, this study investigates whether strain imaging is feasible under these conditions.

5.7.1 Methods

The in vivo experiments were performed with patients' consent during interventional procedures with indicated use of IVUS. The initial study comprised four patients. Rf-data were acquired while examining the left anterior descending artery (LAD) of each patient. 40 MHz transducers were used in combination with a conventional IVUS system (Galaxy, Boston Scientific, USA). The experimental setup described in chapter 5.3 was used for the acquisitions. Consecutive frames were acquired for 3 seconds at a frame rate of $30s^{-1}$ and stored to disk. Simultaneously, an electrocardiogram (ECG) was recorded along with the intraluminal pressure, which was measured with a pressure guide wire (Wavewire, Jomed, USA).

The image sequences were visually inspected for NURD. Images that showed more than one sector of distortion were not considered for strain image calculation. Also, frame pairs that exhibited a mean normalized cross correlation coefficient r_{norm} lower than 0.7 were excluded from further processing. The strain images were calculated offline. One-dimensional radial strain was estimated from consecutive frames with the algorithms described in chapter 3.3. Variations of the blood pressure during the heart cycle yielded the pressure difference required for strain imaging. Segmentation of the luminal borders was performed manually by experts.

After the interventional procedures, reference data were obtained with a PVA phantom. Consecutive images were acquired without intraluminal pressure differences at different degrees of catheter angulation. This was done in order to assess NURD which is specific to the motor and the catheter in use. A NURD evaluation prior to the exam would be desirable, but the catheters are sterile, single-use devices and would be rendered non-sterile after phantom acquisitions.

5.7.2 Results and discussion

The analysis of the acquired image series reveals that the image correlation reaches a maximum during the diastolic phase of the heart cycle. Only during this phase images are sufficiently correlated for strain imaging, because motion artifacts are reduced. During systole, the contraction of the heart and catheter motion render unfeasible the calculation of strain. However, motion is still present even in diastole and often degrades strain estimation results, during a heart cycle only a small number of image frames are suitable for strain analysis.

Figures 5.26 and 5.27 show results from two different patients. B-mode images with 60 dB dynamic range are displayed along with the strain images calculated from two consecutive frames of data. The strain is displayed only in a small area around the luminal border. With increased depth the signal correlation is reduced and strain calculation is not feasible, this area is blackened out. Both positive and negative strains (compression and expansion) are shown. The acquired physiological signals are also shown for a time span of two seconds. The arrow in the pressure plot indicates the acquisition time of the two consecutive data sets. In both presented cases data were acquired during diastole.

The B-mode image in Figure 5.26 shows a shadow at 1 o'clock, which is caused by the guide wire. The image also exhibits a thickened intima with a plaque formation between 2 and 6 o'clock. The strain image shows that parts of this plaque exhibit a high positive strain between 4 and 6 o'clock. The surrounding tissue exhibits areas of low strain. These differences are not visible in the B-mode image.

The B-mode image in Figure 5.27 shows an artery with a larger lumen. The intima appears homogeneous around the circumference. A guide wire artifact is visible at 5 o'clock. The strain image reveals that compression and expansion occur at the same time. Around 6 and 12 o'clock the tissue is compressed, while it expands around 4 and 10 o'clock. A possible explanation is that blood pressure differences are not the only source of compression. Coronary vessels consist of muscular tissue and are located on the epicardial surface of the heart muscle. Muscle contraction introduces additional external vessel deformation. The fact that the areas of compression and expansion are located opposite to each other on the vessel circumference corroborate this hypothesis.

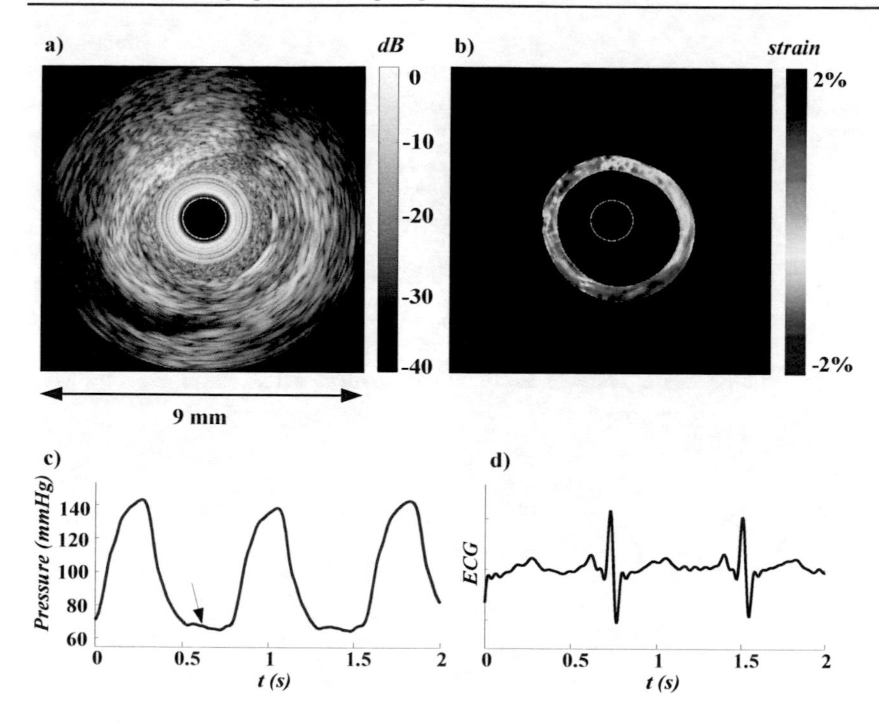

Figure 5.26: B-mode image (a) and corresponding strain image (b) of a coronary artery in vivo, intravascular pressure(c) and ECG (d). The arrow indicates the time of data acquisition.

Visual inspection of the video loops recorded by the IVUS system revealed that NURD with more than two distorted segments occurred in two cases. The artifacts were reduced when repositioning the catheter or examining a different vessel segment. None of the catheters exhibited visible NURD in the subsequent phantom experiments, which were performed with different catheter angulation. This suggests that NURD is not only dependent on the equipment in use, but also is a dynamic phenomenon that is influenced by movement of the heart and the specific vessel anatomy. Sharp catheter bends in combination with dynamic compression are a probable cause of NURD. Thus, it is expected that NURD is less frequent in arteries with moderate tortuosity, e.g. the right coronary artery (RCA) or the LAD.

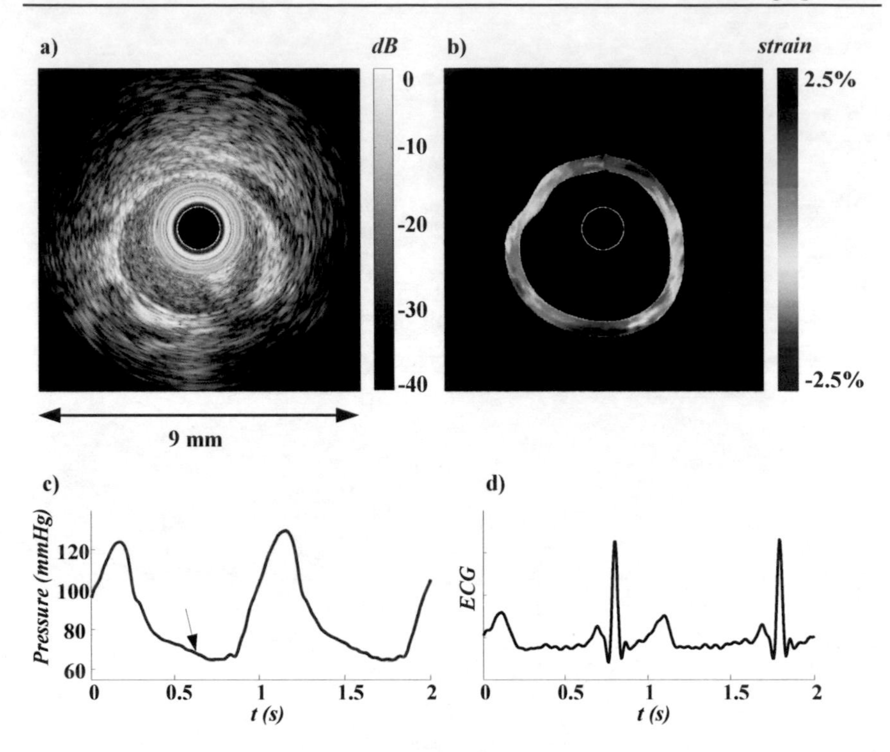

Figure 5.27: B-mode image (a) and corresponding strain image (b) of a coronary artery in vivo, intravascular pressure(c) and ECG (d). The arrow indicates the time of data acquisition.

The applied algorithm estimates radial strain along the A-lines. During a heart cycle the images often show rotational movements of the vessel. The resulting lateral (circumferential) motion in the ultrasound images causes decorrelation and degrades strain estimation results. The application of two dimensional strain estimation concepts is expected to enhance the results to some extend. However, this approach also fails in the presence of speckle decorrelation and out-of-plane motion. Another method for the reduction of motion artifacts is the combination of a catheter with an angioplasty balloon [31]. After inflation the catheter movement within the vessel is prevented, the transducer is also centered within the lumen. However, the use of a balloon for imaging purposes is hardly tolerable for the patient.

In contrast to the phantom experiments with known tissue properties, the presented strain results could not be verified. The examples were chosen based on image correlation and the plausibility of the signal shift and strain results. The only way to verify the results is a study with patients subjected to heart transplant. These patients can be imaged in vivo, histology can be performed after the transplant.

5.7.3 Conclusions

The results of this study show that strain imaging with rotating single element transducers is feasible in vivo. The dependancy of NURD on dynamic compression by the heart muscle has to be investigated in more detail. The image correlation is highest during diastole, but strain image calculation was not possible in all cycles of an image sequence. Lateral motion is present in most data sets. This suggests that the applied strain imaging algorithms should be extended to two dimensions in the future.

5.8 Summary

This chapter presented experimental studies with rotating single element transducers. The transducer characteristics were assessed with respect to axial and lateral resolution. A system for continuous acquisition of rf-data was developed that allows the real-time calculation of strain images with up to 7 frames per second.

Several aspects of NURD were investigated experimentally with phantom studies. No significant relationship was found between catheter angulation and NURD. The degree of NURD rather depends on the mechanical properties of the individual catheters and the motor drive. It was also shown that decorrelation due to NURD can be reduced by beam realignment.

The strain imaging performance of the algorithms presented in chapter 3.3 in conjunction with single element transducers was investigated in vitro and in vivo. It was shown that radial strain imaging is feasible, the results are reproducible under controlled conditions. The in vivo feasibility was also demonstrated. The presence of motion artifacts suggests that more robust algorithms for 2-D strain estimation should be developed for further clinical trials.

6 Segmentation of IVUS images

6.1 Segmentation with deformable models

6.1.1 Introduction

A prerequisite for intracoronary strain imaging is the reliable detection of the luminal border and the discrimination of blood and vessel tissue. Relative strain within the plaque tissue has to be determined, for this task the vessel wall has to be segmented as a starting point. Without this preprocessing step, most strain imaging algorithms yield inaccurate results. Since manual contour tracing is time consuming, automated segmentation is required for clinical evaluation.

Extensive studies have been performed for the development of segmentation algorithms for intravascular ultrasound images in two and three dimensions. Most of these methods require user interaction for contour initialization, some are fully automated. The main goals are the measurement of lumen area and diameter as well as the determination of plaque burden. A major obstacle in this context is caused by the backscatter properties of blood at high frequencies. With IVUS, the frequencies currently range from 20 to 40 MHz. Beyond 20 MHz, the backscatter of blood can approach the same level as backscatter from the vessel wall [109], which makes the segmentation of the lumen difficult. However, flowing blood shows higher variations in the echo pattern than the slowly moving vessel wall. This effect can be used for blood noise reduction and vessel wall detection in several ways. Li et al. proposed temporal averaging of consecutive B-mode images to reduce the echo intensity of blood [100]. Gronningsaeter et al. developed a lateral low pass filter for blood noise suppression [73]. The analysis of high frequency components in the time domain and lateral spatial domain was applied by Takagi et al. [188]. In addition to the application of filter techniques, several groups analyzed the decorrelation properties of blood [74, 75, 102]. Gronnigsaeter et al. analyzed cross correlation estimates from rf-data as well as envelope detected images [74]. The performance was verified with phantom experiments and segmentation was performed by applying a threshold to the correlation estimator. The temporal correlation of blood scattering signals was investigated by Li and co-workers [101]. In their rf-based approach the echo traces were weighted with a function derived from correlation processing, resulting in efficient blood noise reduction. However, all correlation based blood echo suppression methods assume that vessel wall motion is minimal and frame to frame correlation is high in comparison to blood echoes. Often, vessel wall motion can be significant, which leads to decorrelation and causes a blurring effect when frames are averaged [75, 100]. Thus, blood noise reduction should be applied as a preprocessing step in conjunction with other segmentation techniques.

Several groups investigated the use of cost minimizing algorithms and graph searching techniques for IVUS image segmentation. Li et al. developed a semi-automatic 3D segmentation scheme, in which a cost minimizing algorithm was used to identify luminal borders and media-adventitia interfaces in each frame [100]. The node cost was assigned to the spatial first derivative of the image intensity, an optimal path was calculated by dynamic programming techniques. A knowledge based segmentation approach was designed by Sonka and co-workers [178]. They proposed a cost minimizing algorithm incorporating a priori information about the contour shape and features of the echo signals, such as a double echo pattern at the media-adventitia interface. Dijkstra et al. used a similar cost minimizing approach and incorporated the sagittal view of IVUS pullbacks for 3D reconstruction [45]. Takagi et al. applied a gradient based cost minimizing algorithm for the detection of luminal borders and the external elastic membrane [188]. Energy minimizing active contour models (snakes) for segmentation of IVUS images were applied by different groups [92, 95, 108, 116]. Most of these approaches use the image intensity and its gradient as an external image energy. They can be used for the segmentation of several vessel layers, but often require manual interaction and can be computationally complex.

In conjunction with strain imaging the segmentation task is less complex. For strain imaging, only the luminal border has to be segmented as a starting point. Also, only image sequences with highly correlated echo signals from the vessel tissue are selected for strain imaging. This suggests that image correlation can be used as additional information for vessel wall detection. Therefore, in this work the evaluation of correlation properties is combined with the application of deformable models, also often termed active contours. In this chapter, a computationally efficient segmentation method for the detection of the luminal border in IVUS images is developed. This approach uses the frame to frame decorrelation properties of flowing blood to obtain an estimate of the border. Rather than relying on information obtained from single frames alone, this approach evaluates the normalized correlation coefficient of consecutive frames that are selected for strain image processing. The contours are estimated with application of energy minimizing deformable models. The predominant image forces are obtained directly from the correlation coefficient distribution and its gradient. Two algorithms are compared for this task: A dynamic programming approach which searches for a global energy minimum, and a more computationally efficient Greedy algorithm. The former is expected to be more accurate because it is insensitive to local energy minima. The latter is a fast method that searches for the contour by a local minimization of the contour energy [212]. The performance of these algorithms is verified with IVUS data acquired in vivo. The results are compared with contours drawn manually by clinical experts.

6.1.2 Correlation properties of flowing blood

The presence of blood echoes at high frequencies complicates the segmentation of vessel walls [100]. Blood and vessel wall often cannot be reliably distinguished in in IVUS images due to the high level of blood backscatter. Figure 6.1 shows a B-mode image of a coronary vessel as an example. The bright area at the top of the image is the signal ring-down artifact. The blurred area around 100° is presumably caused by NURD. The vessel wall is visible as a slightly brighter area, though the amplitude of blood backscatter is substantial and threshold or gradient based segmentation techniques will fail in many cases. However, the decorrelation properties of flowing blood can be evaluated to obtain additional information for segmentation. During diastole the tissue motion is expected to be low, while the blood flow is reaching its maximum at the same time [72]. Correlation based evaluation of consecutive frames should thus provide significant differences between blood and tissue.

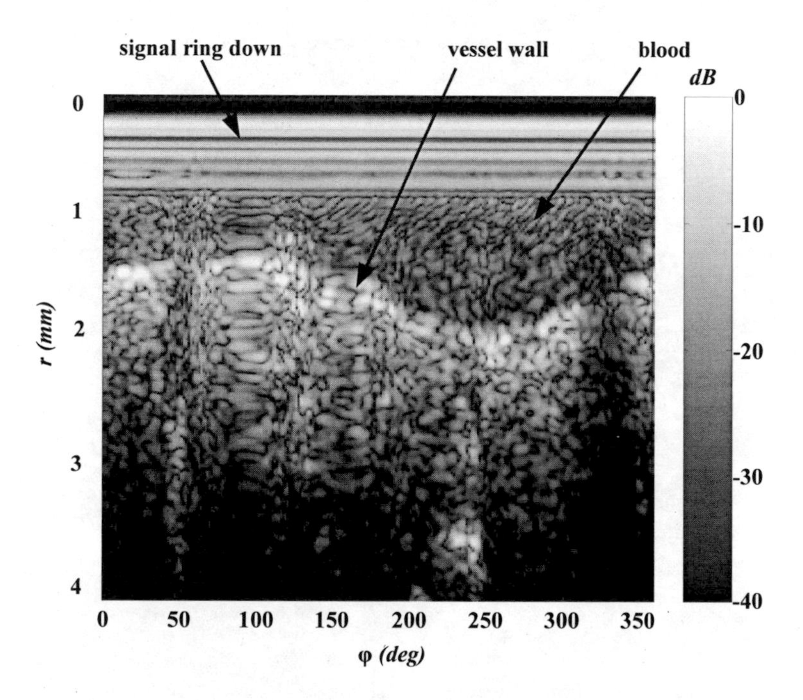

Figure 6.1: B-mode image of a coronary vessel in polar coordinates. The bright area at the top displays the echo signal ring-down.

In order to analyze this effect, the normalized cross correlation coefficient defined in Equation 5.4.2 was evaluated. However, the time shift τ_{k_i} in Equation 5.4.2 was not estimated and set to zero for computational efficiency. Thus, images with the local distribution of the cross correlation coefficient were formed, which is termed $\rho(r,\varphi)$ in the remainder of this chapter. Figure 6.2 shows such an image in polar coordinates, calculated from two consecutive frames. A 2-D median filter with a kernel of 3x3 pixels was applied for smoothing. The upper part of the image shows a highly correlated area, which can be identified as the echo signal ring-down artifact. Below this area a region of low correlation represents the lumen with flowing blood. The vessel wall can be identified as another region of high correlation. From the correlation image an initial contour of the vessel border can be estimated by a simple threshold algorithm with subsequent median filtering of the contour in angular direction. The best results were obtained with a threshold of $\rho=0.7$ and a lateral median filter of 20 pixels for the initial contour. If the threshold was chosen too high, the initial contour deviated from the luminal border, which degraded the segmentation results. The resulting initial contour was used as a priori knowledge for the following segmentation with deformable models.

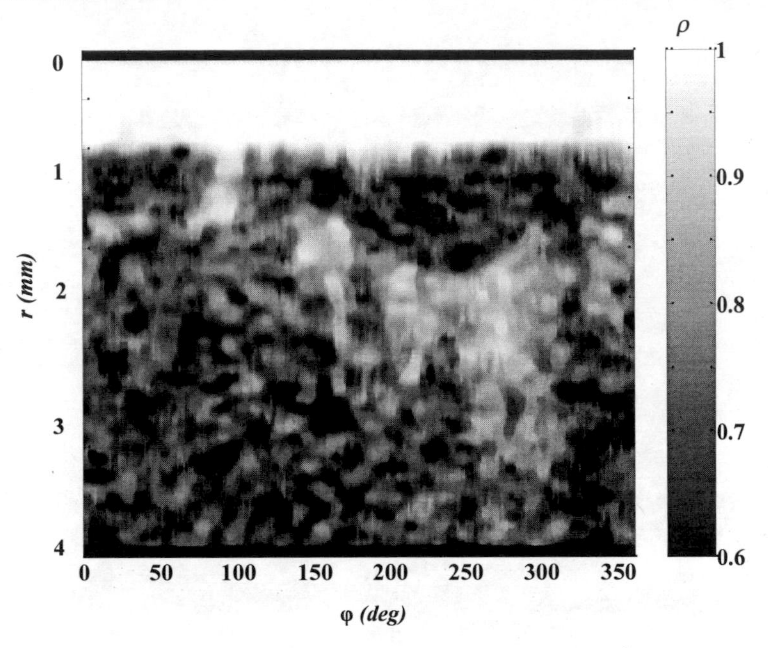

Figure 6.2: Local distribution of the normalized correlation coefficient ρ in polar coordinates. The echo signal ring-down at the top of the image is highly correlated. Flowing blood can be identified as an area of low correlation.

6.1.3 Deformable models

Deformable models are represented by energy minimizing splines under the influence of external image forces. The smoothness of the spline is controlled by internal forces. By minimizing the total energy, an optimal contour is found. In the work of Kass et al. [88] the active contours are termed "snakes" and the energy functional is determined by:

$$E(\mathbf{v})=\int_0^1 (E_{internal}(\mathbf{v}(s))+E_{image}(\mathbf{v}(s))+E_{con}(\mathbf{v}(s)))\,ds \tag{6.1.1}$$

In this equation, the contour is represented by the vector $\boldsymbol{v}(s)$ with arc length s as parameter. $E_{internal}$ represents the contour's internal energy which occurs due to bending. It contains a first and second order derivative term of $\boldsymbol{v}(s)$ which yield high energies in the presence of discontinuities or corners. E_{image} denotes the energy due to image forces, i.e. the image intensity and image gradient magnitude. E_{con} represents external constraint forces that can be user defined to attract contours to specific image features. When discretizing the integral in (6.1.1), the equation can be written as:

$$E(\boldsymbol{v})=\sum_{i=1}^{N} E_{internal}(\boldsymbol{v}_i)+E_{image}(\boldsymbol{v}_i)+E_{con}(\boldsymbol{v}_i) \qquad (6.1.2)$$

Here, $\boldsymbol{v}_i$ denotes the vector to the ith contour point. The discrete internal energy term can be written as [1]:

$$E_{internal}(\boldsymbol{v}_i)=(\alpha_w|\boldsymbol{v}_i-\boldsymbol{v}_{i-1}|^2+\beta_w|\boldsymbol{v}_{i+1}-2\boldsymbol{v}_i+\boldsymbol{v}_{i-1}|^2)/2 \qquad (6.1.3)$$

The terms α_w and β_w are weights to control the contour's continuity and curvature.

In this work, active contour models were adapted to estimate contours in IVUS images. The energy functionals were modified to account for the vessel specific contour geometry. A priori knowledge about the contour was also included. In polar coordinates, the luminal contour will be a more or less smooth, continuous line in circumferential direction, spanning the complete angular range from 0° to 360°. Discrete points on the contour can be written as $\boldsymbol{v}_i=(r(\boldsymbol{v}_i),\varphi(\boldsymbol{v}_i)),\ i=1..N$. The geometry of this setup is outlined in Figure 6.3. For the contour model it is assumed that the circumferential position of the contour points rises monotonically, i.e. $\varphi(\boldsymbol{v}_i)<\varphi(\boldsymbol{v}_{i+1})$ With this assumption, it is feasible to fix angular positions of contour points and allow their movement only in radial direction, where each contour point can move to M different radial positions in a search region. This simplifies the contour search and increases computational efficiency. Another advantage of this approach is that clustering of points due to high image forces is avoided automatically. Also, the contour does not shrink due to internal forces as it would in cartesian coordinates, it rather tends to form a straight line. Finally, with points only moving in radial direction, no sharp corners can be formed. It is thus feasible to omit the second order derivative term (weighted with β_w)in Equation (6.1.3) for further reduction of complexity.

Energy terms representing E_{image} were also selected with respect to computational efficiency and the special segmentation task at hand. The most important image feature considered here is the correlation image $\rho(r,\varphi)$ and its' gradient, since blood and tissue regions show a high contrast in correlation. B-mode image intensity $I(r,\varphi)$ was also used for contour estimation.

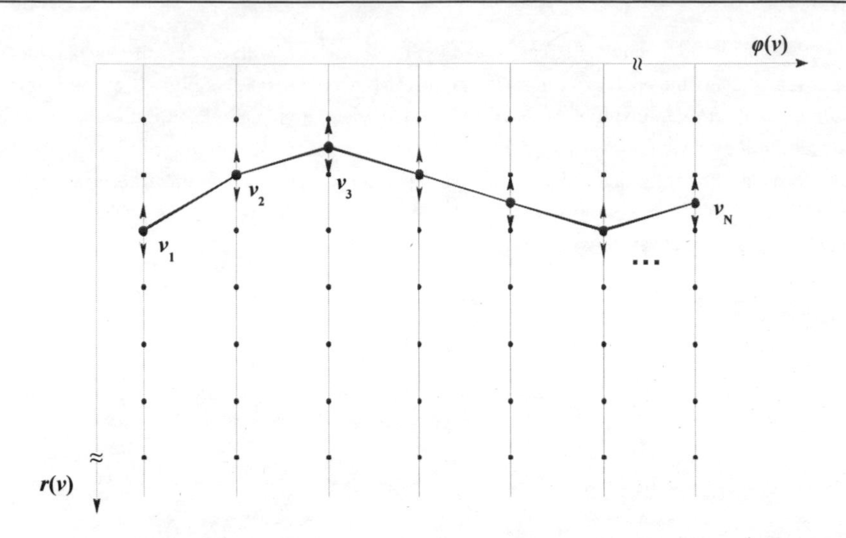

Figure 6.3: Geometry of the discrete contour model in polar coordinates. Contour points are only allowed to move radially along the A-lines.

However, intensity was considered less important and weights were chosen weaker, since contrast between blood and tissue is often poor. For contour estimation the gradient in radial direction (denoted by ∇_r) was computed on both images. Thus, E_{image} can be expressed as:

$$E_{image}(\boldsymbol{v}_i) = -\gamma_w(\nabla_r \cdot \rho(r(\boldsymbol{v}_i), \varphi(\boldsymbol{v}_i))) - \delta_w(|\nabla_r \cdot I(r(\boldsymbol{v}_i), \varphi(\boldsymbol{v}_i))|) \quad (6.1.4)$$

Prior to the calculation of the gradient, the images were filtered with a low pass filter in angular direction to reduce image noise. The gradient images were also normalized to the interval of [0 1], so the weights did not have to be changed for different frames. For this, all negative gradient values of the correlation image were set to zero and the positive values were scaled so that the maximum equals one. This is feasible because the sign of the gradient in the correlation image is known at the vessel wall ($\nabla_r \cdot \rho(r(\boldsymbol{v}_i), \varphi(\boldsymbol{v}_i)) > 0$ for transitions from blood to tissue). Figure 6.4 shows an example of the correlation gradient.

Two external constraint forces were applied in this work. First, an external force was introduced that attracts contour points to the border of the signal ring-down artifact, which can be seen in Figure 6.1. This is necessary for two reasons: On the one hand, the vessel wall is sometimes in contact with the transducer. In those cases the gradient $\nabla_r \cdot \rho(r(\boldsymbol{v}_i), \varphi(\boldsymbol{v}_i))$ is negligible (both artifact and vessel wall show high correlation) and the contour can be attracted to undesired image features. On the other hand, the media-adventitia border of the layered vessel often yields strong image gradients which attract the contour. The second constraint force introduced here was an initial contour, which was calculated by applying a threshold algorithm to the correlation image. Starting at the signal ring-down border, the initial contour was calculated by finding the first location in each A-ine that exceeds a certain correlation magnitude. The contour points are attracted to this initial contour during the search. This is an additional measure to avoid the attraction of the contour to the media-adventitia interface. The energy term E_{con} can thus be expressed as:

$$E_{con}(\mathbf{v}_i)=(\epsilon|\mathbf{v}_i-\mathbf{v}_{ring,i}|^2+\kappa|\mathbf{v}_i-\mathbf{v}_{cont,i}|^2) \quad (6.1.5)$$

Here, $\mathbf{v}_{ring,i}$ and $\mathbf{v}_{cont,i}$ denote the position of the artifact border and the initial contour, respectively. The weights for all energy terms were determined empirically. The same weights were used for all points on the contour.

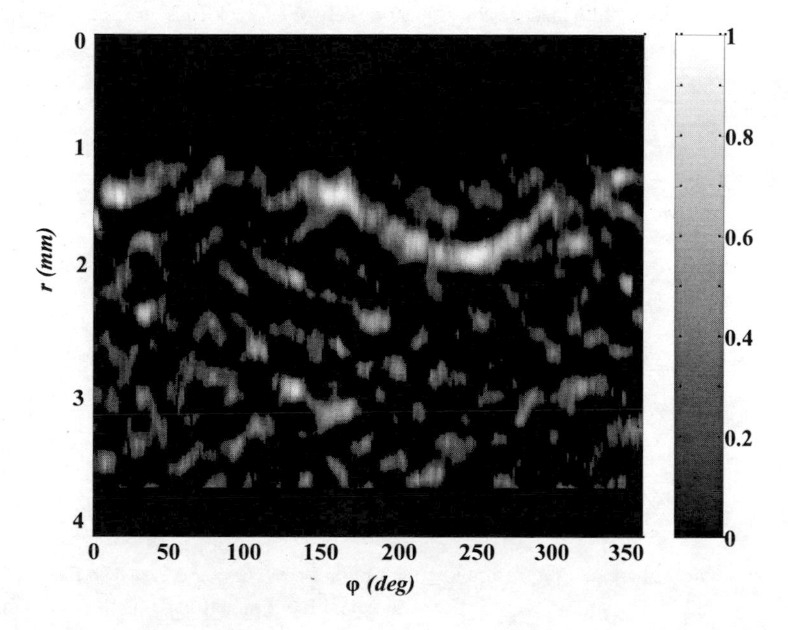

Figure 6.4: Gradient of the normalized correlation coefficient shown in figure 6.2. Only positive gradients (transition from low to high correlation values) are displayed. The vessel border is visible as a bright line.

6.1.4 Dynamic programming algorithm

For the energy minimizing task two algorithms were applied and their performance was compared. In the first algorithm, the contour estimation is represented by a graph searching problem. Each pixel of an image represents a vertex in the graph and is assigned the image energy E_{image}. These vertices are connected by edges, which in turn are assigned the internal energy $E_{internal}$. The graph has N layers, one for each contour point. Each graph layer consists of M vertices, corresponding to a search region of M pixels for every contour point. The task is to find the optimal path through the graph with minimum Energy:

$$E_{min}(\boldsymbol{v}) = \min_{\boldsymbol{v}}[E(\boldsymbol{v})] \tag{6.1.6}$$

A possible solution for finding this optimal path would be an exhaustive search through all possible combinations of paths. However, this is prohibitive because of the high computational cost of the order $O(M^N)$. To reduce complexity, problems of this type can be solved with dynamic programming algorithms [1]. This approach searches for the optimal path by breaking up the function in Equation (6.1.6) into addends and performing the minimization for each addend.

The minimization is performed recursively and can be written as:

$$\begin{aligned}
E_{min,1}(\boldsymbol{v}_1) &= \min_{\boldsymbol{v}_1}[E_{image}(\boldsymbol{v}_1) + E_{cont}(\boldsymbol{v}_1)] \\
E_{min,2}(\boldsymbol{v}_2) &= \min_{\boldsymbol{v}_2}[E_{min,1} + E_{internal}(\boldsymbol{v}_2) + E_{image}(\boldsymbol{v}_2) + E_{cont}(\boldsymbol{v}_2)] \\
&\vdots \\
E_{min,i}(\boldsymbol{v}_i) &= \min_{\boldsymbol{v}_i}[E_{min,i-1}(\boldsymbol{v}_{i-1}) + E_{internal}(\boldsymbol{v}_i) + E_{image}(\boldsymbol{v}_i) + E_{cont}(\boldsymbol{v}_i)] \\
&\vdots \\
E_{min,N}(\boldsymbol{v}_N) &= \min_{\boldsymbol{v}_N}[E_{min,N-1}(\boldsymbol{v}_{N-1}) + E_{internal}(\boldsymbol{v}_N) + E_{image}(\boldsymbol{v}_N) + E_{cont}(\boldsymbol{v}_N)] = E_{min}(\boldsymbol{v})
\end{aligned} \tag{6.1.7}$$

Note that only two neighboring nodes are considered for the calculation of each internal energy, i.e. only the first internal energy term of Equation (6.1.3) is considered:

$$E_{internal}(\boldsymbol{v}_i) = \alpha_w |\boldsymbol{v}_i - \boldsymbol{v}_{i-1}|^2 \tag{6.1.8}$$

For each minimization step the position of the optimal predecessor is stored. After the final step, a global minimum is found. The corresponding optimal path is then found by backtracking through the stored predecessors. This procedure reduces the computational complexity to $O(M \cdot N^2)$. When considering the second internal energy term, the complexity increases to $O(M \cdot N^3)$ and the storage of two predecessors is required for each position [1]. For reasons of computational efficiency this approach was not implemented.

From another point of view, this model could also be considered as a first order Markov process [137, 156]. Such a model consists of a finite number of states that are assigned an individual probability. The probability of switching from one state to the next is described by transition probabilities. The energy minimization problem can be regarded as finding the optimal (most probable) path through a trellis diagram [62] with nodes being states and branches representing transitions. In this particular application, the image and constraint forces represent the state probabilities, while the internal energies denote the transition probabilities. In this first order Markov process, The probability of being in a given state only depends on the preceding state. The algorithm of choice for solving this problem would be the Viterbi algorithm [62], which works similar to the dynamic programming approach described above.

6.1.5 Greedy algorithm

The second algorithm applied in this work is a computationally efficient greedy algorithm similar to the one proposed by Williams and Shah [212]. This approach does not search for a global minimum of the contour, it rather minimizes the energy locally in an iterative manner. For each contour point $\boldsymbol{v}_i$ the energy is minimized individually:

$$E_{min,i}(\boldsymbol{v}_i)=min[E_{internal}(\boldsymbol{v}_i)+E_{image}(\boldsymbol{v}_i)+E_{con}(\boldsymbol{v}_i)]\ ,i=1..N \qquad (6.1.9)$$

This procedure is repeated for all points on the contour until a certain energy level is reached or a maximum number of iterations is exceeded. The drawback of this method is that the contour can be attracted by local image features and thus no global optimum is found. However, the complexity of this approach is reduced to $O(M \cdot N)$, even if both energy terms in equation (6.1.3) were considered. Therefore, this is an attractive method for fast contour detection. For the evaluation of this approach calculations were performed excluding the second energy term in equation (6.1.3).

6.1.6 Clinical study

The in vivo experiments were performed during interventional procedures with indicated use of IVUS. This study comprised three patients, one vessel was scanned per patient. An IVUS scanner (Galaxy, Boston Scientific, USA) was used in conjunction with rotating single element IVUS transducers, operating at 40 MHz. The rf-data were acquired with the experimental setup described in chapter 5.3. Consecutive frames were acquired for three seconds and stored to disk. Data processing was performed offline on a 3 GHz personal computer. The image sequences were visually inspected for NURD. Images that showed more than one sector of distortion were excluded from further processing. The cases where the extended ring-down covered the vessel wall were also excluded. Finally, frame pairs with a mean normalized correlation coefficient ρ lower than 0.7 were excepted, because using the coefficient as a contour energy term yields erroneous results in those cases. Besides that, strain imaging is not feasible with images showing a low correlation.

The contours of the luminal borders were drawn manually by two physicians. Each physician drew the contour sets twice in order to obtain also an estimate of intra-observer variance. A time span of four days passed between the drawing of the sets. The segmentation was performed with an interface which allowed the direct comparison with contour point locations obtained from automated segmentation. For evaluation, the mean differences of contours and the corresponding standard deviations were calculated. Results were obtained for inter- and intra-observer differences, as well as for comparisons with the segmentation algorithms.

6.1.7 Segmentation results

A total number of 50 frame pairs were evaluated with the automated segmentation algorithms and compared to manual drawings. The greedy algorithm yielded sufficient results after two iterations, i.e. each contour point was moved twice. The average calculating time for the segmentation (excluding image correlation) was 1.8 s for the greedy algorithm and 2.7 s for the dynamic programming algorithm using a 3 GHz processor.

Segmentation results of two different patients are exemplarily shown in polar coordinates in Figure 6.5. The image a) is the same as the one in Figure 6.1. The white lines represent manually drawn contours, while the black lines show contours obtained with the two algorithms. Both images exhibit a guide wire artifact which is visible as a dark region around 320°. At this location the vessel wall is more difficult to detect and the contours deviate. The left image exhibits a region of NURD around 100°. In this region the contours also deviate. A possible explanation for this effect is that blood correlation is higher in this area and thus no significant correlation gradient is present (see also Figures 6.2 and 6.4).

An overview of the segmentation results is given in Table 6.1. The differences of contour radii are presented as mean values and standard deviations. For each contour 256 angular positions were considered. Inter- and intra-observer differences were evaluated as well as a comparison between manually drawn contours and algorithms. The last column shows differences between the two segmentation algorithms. The size of an image pixel in radial direction was 7.8 μm (e.g. The 0.05 mm intra-observer standard deviation of expert A corresponds to 6.4 pixels).

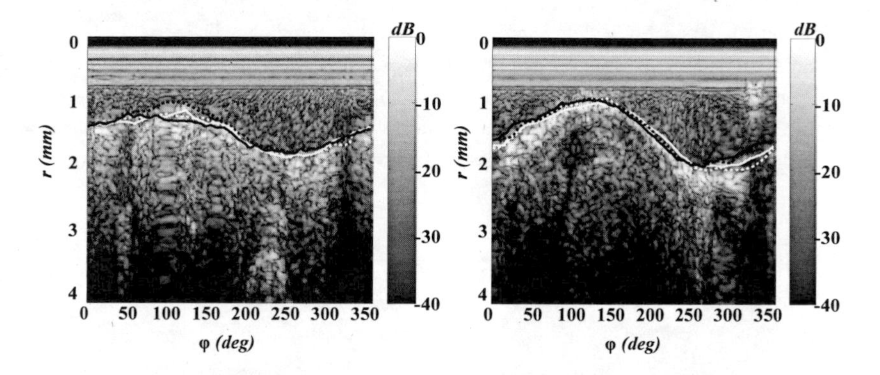

Figure 6.5: Two B-mode images in polar coordinates with segmentation results of observer 1 (white dashed line), observer 2 (white solid line), dynamic programming algorithm (black dashed line), and greedy algorithm (black solid line).

difference of contours	**A-A**	**A-B**	**B-B**	**A-D**	**A-G**	**B-D**	**B-G**	**D-G**
μ (mm)	0.021	-0.027	0.009	0.038	0.011	0.065	0.038	-0.027
σ (mm)	0.050	0.100	0.066	0.085	0.117	0.085	0.124	0.097

Table 6.1: Mean and standard deviation of differences in radial contour positions. The columns 2 to 4 show inter- and intra-observer differences of human experts A and B. In columns 5 to 8 a comparison of manually drawn contours to the greedy algorithm (G) and the dynamic programming approach (D) is given. Column 9 presents the differences between both algorithms.

The Figures 6.6 and 6.7 give a more detailed overview of the segmentation results. The data are presented as Bland-Altman plots, where the contour differences are plotted versus their mean values. Figure 6.6 shows a comparison of manually drawn contours with the two algorithms. The greedy algorithm yields higher standard deviations than the dynamic programming approach. The plots on the right side also show a linear trend for small contour radii (around 1.5 mm). A possible explanation is that the greedy algorithm exhibits erroneous results in the vicinity of the ring down. This effect is less prominent with the dynamic programming approach. Figure 6.7 shows the intra- and inter-observer results. The intra-observer results yield the lowest standard deviations. However, the inter-observer differences are higher, they are comparable to the plots in Figure 6.6. The lower right plot in Figure 6.7 shows the deviations of the two algorithms, which are on the same order as the inter-observer differences.

A variation of the energy weights shows that the cross correlation image is an important feature for energy minimization. When the corresponding weights are reduced or set to zero, the segmentation performance severely degrades. In those cases the contour is often attracted by image gradients at the media-adventitia interface, which is exemplarily shown in cartesian coordinates in Figure 6.8. Here, the black contour was calculated using the correlation image features, while the white contour was obtained with B-mode image features only.

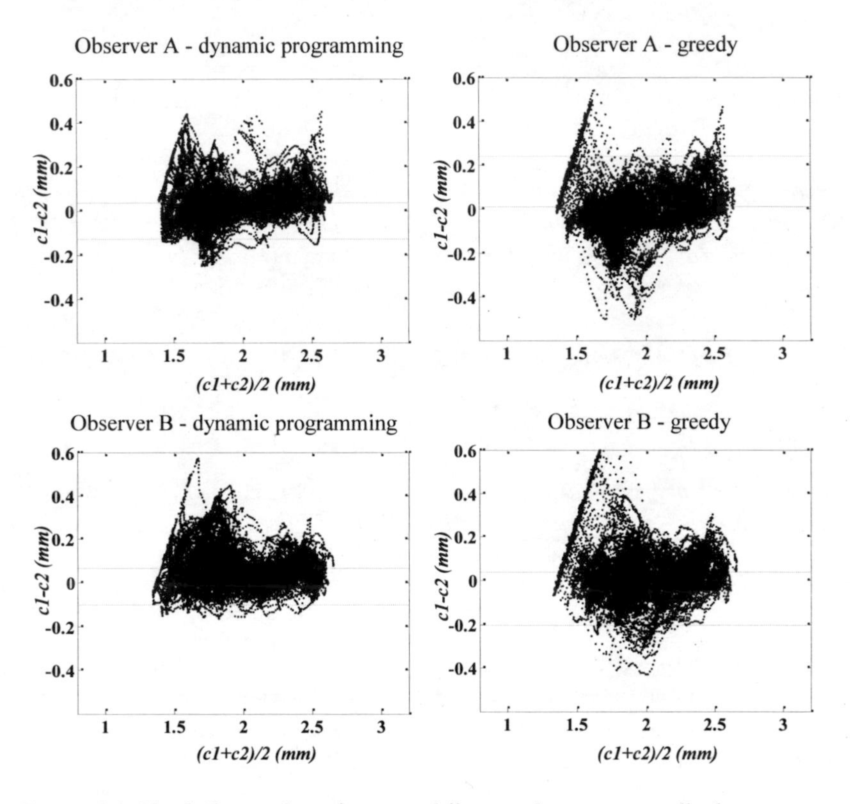

Figure 6.6: Bland-Altman plots of contour differences between manually drawn contours and automated algorithms. The differences of contour points (c1-c2) is plotted versus their mean value. The solid line represents the mean value of differences, the dashed lines denote ± 1.96 standard deviations.

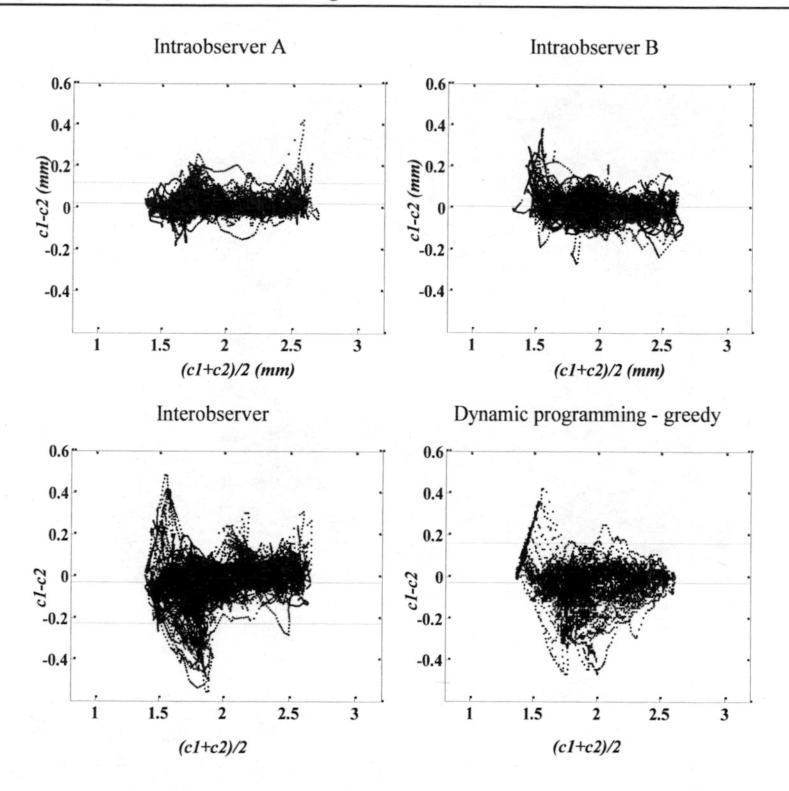

Figure 6.7: Bland-Altman plots of intra- and inter-observer contour differences and differences between the applied algorithms. The differences of contour points (c1-c2) are plotted versus their mean value. The solid line represents the mean value of differences, the dashed lines denote ± 1.96 standard deviations.

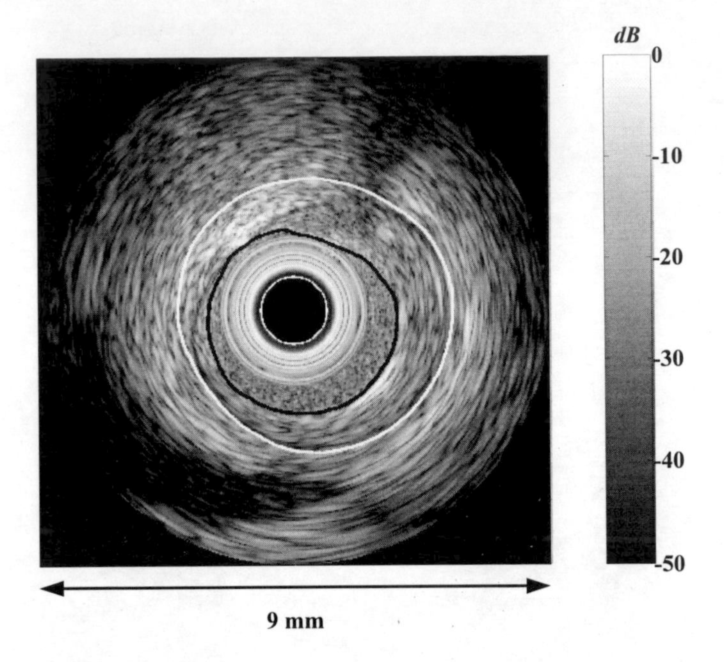

Figure 6.8: B-mode image in cartesian coordinates. The displayed contours were calculated with the dynamic programming algorithm. For the white contour the correlation information was omitted, which leads to an erroneous segmentation of the media-adventitia interface.

6.1.8 Conclusions

The segmentation results show that both analyzed algorithms can be successfully applied for the segmentation of blood and vessel walls. In comparison to manually drawn contours, the standard deviations of the dynamic programming algorithm are lower than those of inter-observer differences. As expected, the contours detected by the greedy algorithm exhibit slightly higher standard deviations in comparison to contours drawn by experts. The variation in manually drawn contours illustrates the advantages of algorithms for automated segmentation with reproducible results for a given parameter set. The dynamic programming approach yields more accurate results because it searches for a global optimum instead of a local energy minimum. However, the applied greedy algorithm delivers sufficient results and is computationally less complex. The erroneous behavior of the greedy algorithm at small contour radii might be related to the proximity of the extended ring-down artifact and has to be investigated further.

The segmentation of images in polar coordinates allows an efficient implementation of the algorithms. Since the angular positions of contour points are fixed, clustering of points is automatically avoided. The variation of image weights corroborate the hypothesis that the correlation coefficient is a prominent image feature. The backscatter of blood at 40 MHz degrades the segmentation results when relying on single B-mode image features alone. The media-adventitia interface often yields a high B-mode image gradient which attracts the contours. In the case of Figure 6.8 this interface is segmented because correlation image information was neglected. This implies that the presented algorithms can also potentially be used for the segmentation of the media-adventitia interface. However, for accurate results additional image features have to be evaluated.

The automated segmentation is not optimized for speed yet. The calculation time for each contour is less than three seconds for both algorithms. However, the low computational complexity especially of the Greedy algorithm suggests that it can be used for a real-time implementation. Also, in the current implementation a contour point was placed on each angular position. For faster computation the number of points could be reduced followed by contour interpolation.

The algorithms analyzed in this chapter were designed to be used in conjunction with strain image processing and depend on high image correlation, which only occurs in certain phases of the heart cycle. For the segmentation of image sequences of a complete heart cycle more complex approaches have to be considered. For instance, a contour persistence or the evaluation of additional image energies will enhance segmentation results. Another promising tool is the additional analysis of textual and spectral information, which will be presented in the next section.

6.2 Segmentation based on textural and spectral information

6.2.1 Introduction

The main advantage of the active contours segmentation algorithms presented in the previous section is their computational efficiency. However, in some cases the segmentation can be erroneous and more advanced algorithms are required. The evaluation of additional ultrasound signal properties such as spectral or textural information was shown to be a promising tool for the characterization and segmentation of tissue [105, 106, 119]. Methods for ultrasonic tissue characterization have been developed for several organs, such as the eye [105], liver [107, 197] and prostate [57, 168, 172]. These methods are usually combined with classification schemes such as neural networks [57] or neuro-fuzzy inference systems [169]. The characterization of plaques with ultrasound has been investigated by several groups. The aim is to identify plaques that are at risk of rupture and cause acute myocardial infarction. Videodensitometry of gray scale images has been proposed [193]. However, the accuracy of this method is limited [120]. The analysis of spectral echo characteristics was shown to be promising. Typical spectral parameters used for evaluation are integrated attenuation and slope of attenuation [16, 213], integrated backscatter [93], y-intercept and midband fit of regression lines [123]. Spectral analysis has also been explored with IVUS [115, 171, 180]. In an in vitro study with post mortem coronary arteries, Moore et al. acquired IVUS rf-data and evaluated several spectral parameters [120]. They performed histologic analysis on the vessel specimens and used the results as a gold standard for comparison. In a refined study the same group divided the tissue into three subgroups and applied a Mahalanobis classifier for discrimination, yielding classification rates of 83% [208]. In a similar approach, Nair et al. used IVUS rf-data for the characterization of coronary plaques [123, 124]. They evaluated spectral characteristics with Fourier transforms and autoregressive processes and categorized plaque tissue with classification trees. Histology was performed for comparison and the tissue was divided into four subgroups. Classification rates ranged from 80% to 90% for the different tissue types.

Textural information has also been evaluated for plaque characterization. Rakebrandt et al. analyzed the texture of ultrasound images of carotid arteries in an in vitro study [157]. A total number of 157 textural analysis algorithms was applied in this study. Christodoulou et al. acquired ultrasound data from carotid vessel specimens and analyzed the data with first and second order statistics [32]. Classification was performed in this study with a neural network. Zhang and coworkers performed texture analysis of IVUS video data and divided the tissue into three classes [217]. The combination of integrated backscatter analysis with textural features for coronary plaque characterization with IVUS was reported by Komiyama et al. [93].

Most of the studies cited above were designed for the discrimination of different plaque types. They included extensive in vitro experiments with histologic analysis, which is beyond the scope of this work. The aim of the study described in this section is the application of tissue characterization algorithms for the discrimination of blood and vessel tissue and the segmentation of the inner vessel wall. This approach is an alternative to the segmentation with active contour models presented in the previous section. The results are expected to be more consistent due to the evaluation of multiple parameters. However, parameter extraction in combination with classification significantly raises the computational cost.

The combined evaluation of spectral features of rf-data and textural information was shown to be a promising approach and yields better classification results than texture information alone [169]. Therefore, spectral parameters as well as first and second order texture parameters were evaluated in this work based on in vivo acquisitions of IVUS rf-data [146]. Tissue describing parameters were estimated directly from rf-data after dividing each rf-frame into numerous ROIs to allow spatially resolved classification. Parameters originating from different parameter groups were compared with each other and a neuro-fuzzy inference system 169] was trained on up to eight parameters to distinguish blood from tissue using a multi-feature approach.

6.2.2 Data acquisition and processing

In vivo acquisitions were performed in the catheter laboratory during interventional procedures. The study currently comprises data sets from four patients. Data were acquired as described in chapter 6.1.6. Consecutive rf-frames were acquired and stored for offline processing. Each frame consists of 256 A-lines. Each line comprises 512 samples, which corresponds to a scan depth of approximately 4 mm. The point spread function of the transducer was determined for spectrum normalization. For this task, images of an acrylic glass plate acting as a specular reflector were acquired as described in chapter 5.2.1. Ten frames were evaluated for each patient, resulting in a total number of 40 data sets. The individual rf- frames were divided into 1386 overlapping ROIs. Each ROI consists of $N=8$ beam lines, where each line comprises $M=64$ samples. The overlap of the ROIs was 75 % in radial and 50 % in circumferential direction.

For the evaluation of spectral features, the data in all ROIs were windowed with a Hamming window and transformed to frequency domain using the FFT. The squared magnitude spectra of all lines in an ROI were then averaged and log compressed. An established analysis method is the linear regression line fit to the power spectrum [106, 115, 123]. From this line, the following spectral parameters were calculated: Mid band value, axis intercept, slope, and square deviation of the linear regression fit to the estimated spectrum of the backscattered signal. These parameters are described in detail in [170].

For the evaluation of textural parameters the data were demodulated using the Hilbert transform. Texture parameters of first and second order were calculated. First order parameters only evaluate the characteristics of individual pixels, while second order texture parameters incorporate the spatial relationship of adjacent pixels. First order texture parameters analyzed in this approach are: Maximum, minimum, mean value, signal to noise ratio (SNR), contrast, full width at half maximum (FWHM), skewness and entropy of the intensity histogram. Texture parameters of second order were estimated after calculation of co-occurrence matrices [179] in radial direction. Second order texture parameters evaluated in this approach are: Angular second moment, contrast, correlation, dimension, entropy, inverse difference moment, kappa and peak density [81, 170].

6.2.3 Fuzzy inference system

The classification approach applied in this work is based on a first order Sugeno-type system and uses Gaussian membership functions to model the underlying parameter distribution [186, 168]. Classification is realized by an adaptive fuzzy inference system which classifies the ROIs into two groups: Blood and vessel tissue.

The system was trained using manual segmentation results drawn by experts as gold standard. Still images as well as video sequences were evaluated during the segmentation process. The number of parameters, the parameters themselves and the number of rules applied to model the parameter distributions are chosen automatically by the system during the training procedure. Spectral and textural parameters are equally considered. The training was performed using four-fold cross validation over patient data sets. Eight parameters and up to five rules are used in this approach. After classification by the fuzzy inference system, a post-processing procedure for the evaluation of contextual information is used to conjoin adjacent ROIs comprising the same tissue properties.

6.2.4 Segmentation results

The parameters yielding the best performance in this study were taken from the group of spectral backscatter features and from the groups of texture parameters of first and second order. From those parameters mentioned in section 6.2.2, the following eight parameters were selected by the system:
- Mid band value, axis intercept (spectral parameters)
- Minimum (MIN), skewness (SKEW), signal to noise ratio (SNR) (first order texture parameters)
- Kappa (KAP), dimension (DIM), contrast (CON) (second order texture parameters).

For completeness, the definitions for the texture parameters are given below. The variable $b_{n,m}$ denotes the amplitude of the demodulated image at sample *m* and line *n* of an ROI of size $M\,x\,N$. The variable $P_{d,n}(i,j)$ represents the co-occurrence matrix [178]. This square matrix describes how frequently two pixels with discrete amplitudes $(i,j)\in 1..N_g$ appear in the ROI separated by distance *d* in line *n*. Since the lateral resolution changes over depth in a circular scan, only distances in radial direction were evaluated for each line.

$$MIN=\frac{1}{N}\sum_{n=1}^{N}\min_{m}(b_{n,m}) \tag{6.2.1}$$

$$SKEW=\frac{1}{N}\sum_{n=1}^{N}\frac{\frac{1}{M}\sum_{m=1}^{M}\left(b_{n,m}-\frac{1}{M}\sum_{m=1}^{M}b_{n,m}\right)^{3}}{\left(\frac{1}{M}\sum_{m=1}^{M}\left(b_{n,m}-\frac{1}{M}\sum_{m=1}^{M}b_{n,m}\right)^{2}\right)^{\frac{3}{2}}} \tag{6.2.2}$$

$$SNR=\frac{1}{N}\sum_{n=1}^{N}\frac{\frac{1}{M}\sum_{m=1}^{M}(b_{n,m})}{\sqrt{\frac{1}{M}\sum_{m=1}^{M}\left(b_{n,m}-\frac{1}{M}\sum_{m=1}^{M}b_{n,m}\right)^{2}}} \tag{6.2.3}$$

$$CON=\frac{1}{N}\sum_{n=1}^{N}\sum_{i=1}^{Ng}\sum_{j=1}^{Ng}|i-j|^{2}P_{d,n}(i,j) \tag{6.2.4}$$

$$DIM = \frac{1}{N}\sum_{n=1}^{N}\frac{1}{g}\sum_{l=0}^{g-1}\sum_{i=1}^{Ng}\sum_{j=1}^{Ng}\frac{P_{d,n}(i,j)}{1+((i-1)-(j-1))^2}\bigg|_{i\neq j}\cdot l^2\big|_{i-j=l} \quad (6.2.5)$$

$$KAP = \frac{1}{N}\sum_{n=1}^{N}\sum_{i=1}^{Ng}\sum_{j=1}^{Ng}\frac{P_{d,n}(i,j)|_{i=j} - P_{d,n}(i,j)\cdot P_{d,n}(j,i)}{P_{d,n}(i,j)|_{i=j} - \min_{i,j}\left\{P_{d,n}(i,j), P_{d,n}(j,i)\right\}} \quad (6.2.6)$$

The classification system yields a fuzzy value for each ROI of the processed frames [170]. Figure 6.9 shows the probabilities of the fuzzy output values to belong to the target groups 'blood' or 'tissue', respectively. In more detail, each ROI was identified as 'blood' or 'tissue' based on the results of manual segmentation. The relative frequency for each output value to belong to one of the target groups was then calculated.

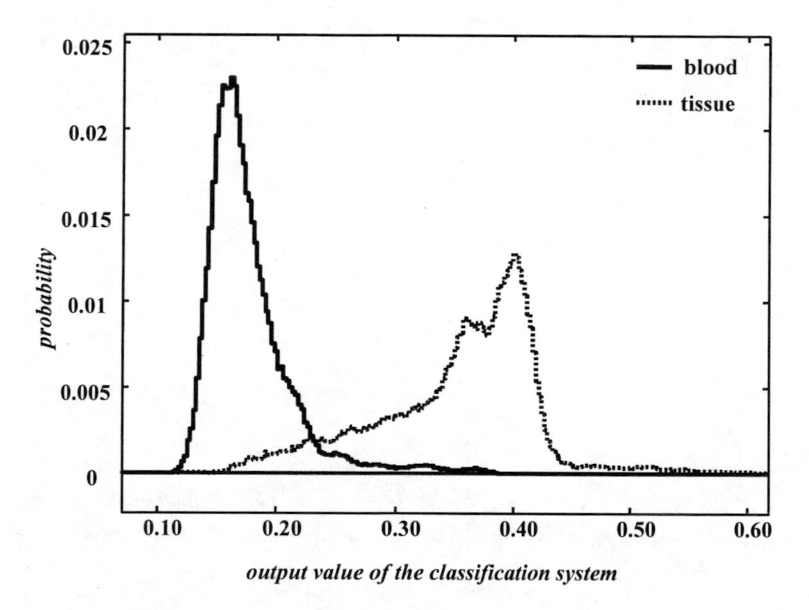

Figure 6.9: Distributions of probabilities of output values to belong to target groups 'blood' or 'tissue'

The output of the fuzzy inference system is a continuous value. A separation threshold for calculation of sensitivity and specificity can thus be chosen from the complete range of values. The left plot in Figure 6.10 shows sensitivity (solid line) and specificity (dotted line) as functions of the separation threshold. The plot on the right side of Figure 6.10 displays the receiver operating characteristic (ROC) curve [168] constructed by plotting sensitivity against specificity. The area under the curve is obtained by varying the separation threshold (abscissa in the left plot). This area comprises a mean value of A_{ROC}=0.95 when estimated using four-fold cross validation over patient data sets.

As an example, Figure 6.11 displays segmentation results of a data set evaluated in this approach. The dynamic range of the plotted images is 60 dB. Between six and eight o'clock calcified plaque is visible, which can be identified by increased echogenicity followed by an acoustic shadow. The black line in the left diagram represents a manually drawn contour of the lumen border. In the right image of Figure 6.11, the appropriate output map of the classification system is shown superimposed over the B-mode image. The overlaid area shows the ROIs classified as blood. The area is contiguous except for a small region at three o'clock which was falsely classified as tissue. When compared to the manually drawn contour, the classification algorithm slightly overestimates the blood region. This effect can be seen at one o'clock and at 6 o'clock.

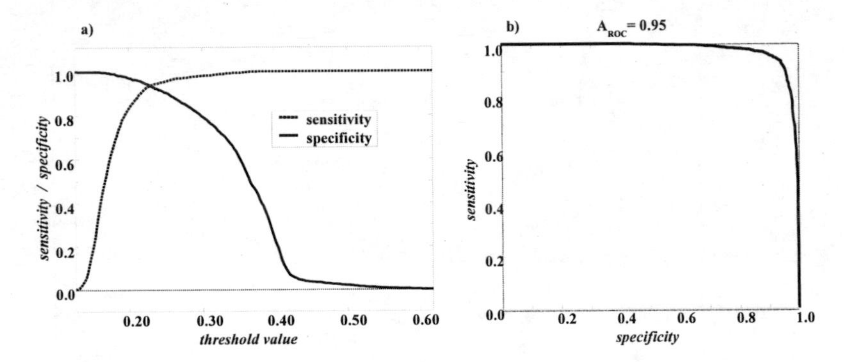

Figure 6.10: Results for the discrimination of blood and tissue. Left: Sensitivity and specificity plotted versus the separation threshold. Right: Sensitivity plotted versus specificity for varying separation thresholds. The area under the ROC curve is A_{ROC} = 0.95 ± 0.02.

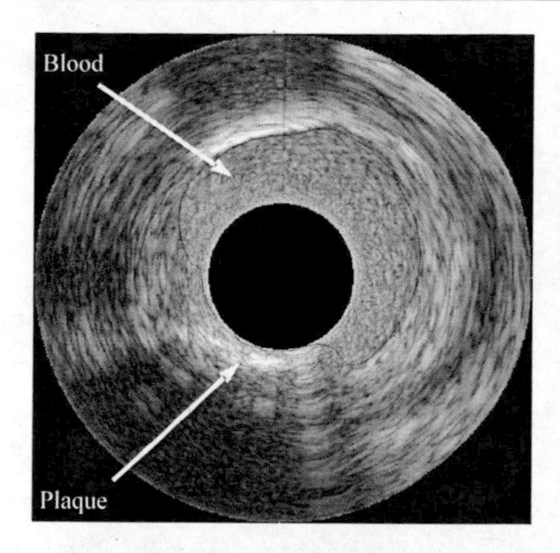

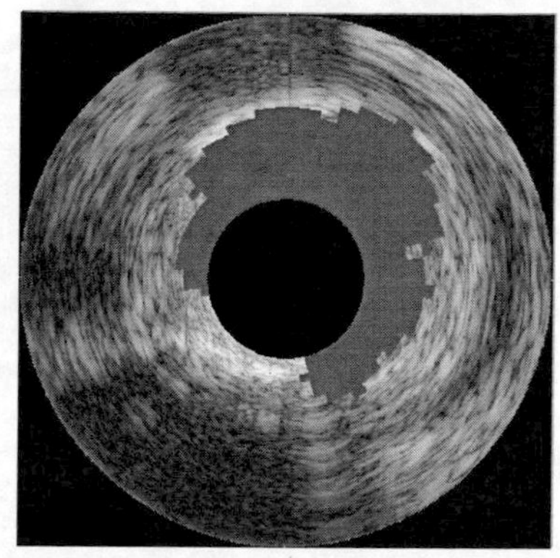

Figure 6.11: Segmentation results. Left: B-mode image of a coronary artery. The black line represents a manually drawn contour. Right: B-mode image with superimposed output of the classification system.

6.2.5 Conclusions

The results show that ROIs belonging to one of the two target groups, blood or tissue, can be successfully classified using the proposed fuzzy inference system. The probability curves in Figure 6.9 exhibit only a small overlapping region. The area under the ROC curve of $A_{ROC}=0.95$ suggests that the two groups can be discriminated with sufficient accuracy.

There is a satisfying agreement when comparing the blood area of the manual segmentation data with the classification results shown in Figure 6.11. Nearly all ROIs of the vessel tissue are classified correctly, including the areas which exhibit acoustic shadowing. The area classified as blood hardly contains gaps, because contextual information about adjacent ROIs is incorporated in a post-processing step [168]. However, the blood area tends to be overestimated at the borders, which might be ascribed to the post-processing routine as well.

The classification rates seem high compared to other tissue characterization methods [208, 217]. However, the classification into only two target groups simplifies the task. Also, data from blood and tissue have distinct spectral and textural features [109, 155] that can well be identified. In more complex classification tasks such as the characterization of different plaque types, the classification rates are expected to be lower.

The main goal of the presented approach is the automated segmentation of blood and tissue. Compared to other segmentation methods such as active contours or random field models, the application of tissue characterization algorithms and the training of a fuzzy inference system are complex and computationally intensive. However, model based methods are often semi-automatic and need an initial contour seed. Once the fuzzy inference system is trained, no user interaction is required. The computationally intensive part is the training phase of the system. After this procedure, the results of several frames can be obtained with calculation times in the order of minutes.

In order to enhance segmentation results, the proposed method could be combined with segmentation algorithms based on deformable models. The output map shown in Figure 6.11 could be used as an initial guess for a luminal contour, which would subsequently be refined with the deformable model. It is expected that this additional step will improve segmentation results in the cases where the luminal area is overestimated.

6.3 Summary

An important preprocessing step for strain imaging is the reliable segmentation of blood and vessel walls in IVUS images. This chapter presented two approaches for vessel wall segmentation. First, a computationally efficient segmentation method for the detection of luminal borders was developed based on deformable models. The frame to frame decorrelation properties of flowing blood were evaluated for vessel wall detection. The normalized correlation coefficient of consecutive frames and its gradient were directly used as image forces for the energy minimizing deformable models. Two algorithms were implemented and compared: A dynamic programming approach and a greedy algorithm which minimizes contour energies locally. Their performance was verified with IVUS data acquired in vivo and compared to contours drawn manually by clinical experts. The results show a good agreement of manually and automatically segmented contours. The evaluation of correlation properties significantly enhances segmentation results.

The second presented method allowed fully automated segmentation of blood and vessel tissue based on the evaluation of spectral and textural image features. The parameters were evaluated and classified using a fuzzy inference system, which was trained and validated with 40 data sets from 4 patients. The system reached classification rates with a mean area under the ROC curve of $A_{ROC}=0.95$ when estimated using four-fold cross validation over patient data sets. ROIs containing blood were determined with high accuracy.

Both methods were successfully applied for vessel wall segmentation, though their performance is not equivalent. The first approach based on deformable models requires no training, is computationally efficient and therefore the preferred method for time critical applications. However, weights have to be carefully chosen and the performance relies on an accurate initial contour, which may require user interaction in some cases. The second approach on the other hand is fully automated and yields high accuracy due to the evaluation of multiple image features. It is the method of choice for cases where accuracy is more relevant than computational time efficiency. But a limiting factor of this approach is the required gold standard data base and the system training phase. These factors have to be taken into account when selecting the appropriate segmentation method for the task at hand.

7 Combined pressure and flow velocity measurements

7.1 Introduction

The main focus of the previous chapters was on intravascular strain imaging aimed at the detection of vulnerable plaques. This chapter deals with the assessment of stable coronary plaques which form stenotic lesions. In clinical practice, many patients are treated who suffer from heart disease caused by arterial narrowing. The severity of coronary stenoses is usually assessed invasively by morphological measurements, such as quantitative coronary angiography (QCA) or intravascular ultrasound (IVUS). However, information about plaque morphology and composition cannot always determine the hemodynamic significance of a stenosis [104]. Angiographic analysis strongly depends on the projection angle and the results are often difficult to interpret. Also, coronary flow at resting conditions remains unchanged with arterial narrowing of up to 75% area stenosis [72]. Besides morphology, information about the hemodynamic significance of a stenosis should be evaluated for diagnosis and treatment planning.

The recent development of guide wires with miniaturized sensor tips allows the evaluation of additional functional information, namely intracoronary pressure and flow velocity. Various methods have been developed for this task, such as the calculation of myocardial fractional flow reserve (FFR) derived from pressure measurements [152] or coronary flow velocity reserve (CFVR), calculated from Doppler flow measurements [72]. Currently, these functional parameters are only assessed separately in clinical practice and the validity of the measurements depends on a state of maximum flow (maximum hyperemia) [154], which cannot be reached in some cases. A pressure based parameter that does not require hyperemia was developed by Brosh et al., evaluating high frequency signal components [18].

The functional significance or resistance of a coronary stenosis can be described more accurately by simultaneous measurement of intracoronary blood flow and the pressure difference caused by the obstruction [72, 117]. Measurements of flow-pressure relationships have been performed in animals [70, 71] and in patients [12, 113, 145]. A prototype wire for combined pressure and flow measurements has been developed and tested in an initial study [176]. However, simultaneous measurements have not been used in clinical routine so far, because two sensor wires were needed and the evaluation of the combined measurements is not standardized yet and usually requires manual editing.

The aim of the study presented in this chapter is twofold: First, the verification of an evaluation procedure for combined pressure and flow measurements that is feasible for clinical practice and yields information about stenosis resistance. Second, the development of a robust pressure based parameter which is independent of maximum hyperemia and can complement the information obtained with FFR in those cases where flow measurements are not feasible. This is done by evaluating the coherence of pressure signals acquired proximal and distal of the lesions.

7.2 Methods

The measurements were performed with informed patients' consent during routine procedures in the catheter lab. 20 patients who were scheduled for diagnostic catheterization or interventional procedures were selected for this trial, a total number of 24 data sets was recorded.

During the catheterization procedure, the aortic pressure p_a proximal of a coronary stenosis was measured using a fluid filled guiding catheter. Pressure guide wires (Radi pressure wire, Radi, Sweden and Wavewire, Jomed, USA) were used for measuring the pressure p_d distal of a lesion. Prior to the examinations the sensor of the pressure wire was placed near the outlet of the guiding catheter and the two pressure signals were equalized to avoid a signal offset. After calibration, the sensor was placed distal to the lesion. For flow velocity measurements, a Doppler guide wire (Flowire, Jomed, USA) was also placed distal to the lesion in the vicinity of the pressure sensor. Figure 7.1 shows a schematic of the measurement setup. Maximum hyperemia was induced by intravenous infusion of 140 µg/kg/min adenosine. Thus, at hyperemia a pressure difference $\Delta p = p_a - p_d$ occurs in the presence of a stenosis.

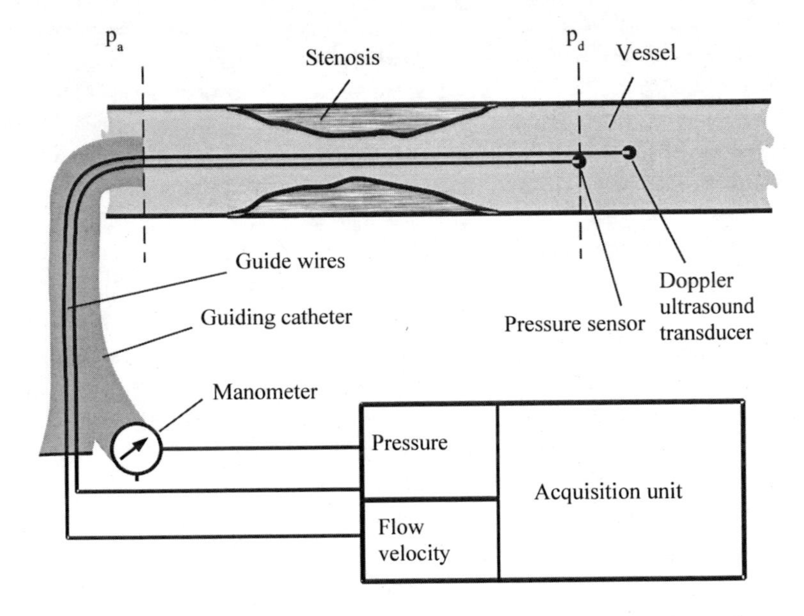

Figure 7.1: Measurement setup for intracoronary pressure and flow velocity signals.

Over a period of two minutes the two pressure signals and the flow velocity were recorded simultaneously, along with an electrocardiogram (ECG). A typical set of signals is shown in Figure 7.2 for a duration of two seconds. The data were digitized at 200 Hz with a 4 channel

A/D converter (ME2000, Meilhaus, Germany) and stored on a personal computer for offline processing. Prior to the analysis the data was low pass filtered (cutoff frequency 20 Hz) to remove unwanted noise.

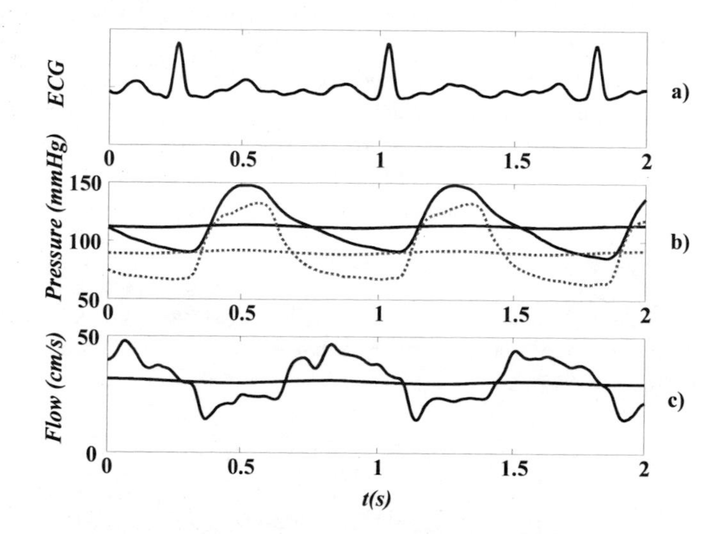

Figure 7.2: Typical data sets consisting of (a) ECG signal, (b) proximal (solid line) and distal (dashed line) pressure signals and (c) flow velocity, shown for two heart cycles. Mean values of pressure and flow velocity calculated with a moving average filter over two heart cycles are also displayed for each signal.

7.2.1 Flow-Pressure relationship

The mean values of pressure and flow velocity were evaluated for the combined analysis. A moving average filter was used to compute average pressure and flow signals. For each patient, a time window of approximately 30 to 60 seconds was selected visually for data analysis. In this time window the intracoronary flow changed from resting conditions to intermediate flow and maximum hyperemia. The different flow conditions in this time window are illustrated in Figure 7.3. Here, the pressure and flow velocity waveforms and their mean values are plotted. The flow is minimal at rest and reaches a maximum at hyperemia. The increase of the mean pressure difference clearly indicates the presence of a stenosis.

In [72, 113] it was shown that the relationship of flow and pressure difference in the presence of a stenosis can be approximated by a 2nd order polynomial equation derived from fluid dynamics in rigid tubes:

$$\Delta p = a \cdot V + b \cdot V^2 \tag{7.2.1}$$

Here, Δp denotes the pressure difference and V denotes the flow velocity. The values a and b are constants that have to be determined for stenosis characterization. However, this evaluation is usually performed in certain parts of the heart cycle [72], which requires manual selection of signal windows for each cycle. This approach is time consuming and might not be feasible in clinical practice. Therefore, in this work the average pressure difference $\Delta \bar{p}$ was plotted against average flow velocity $\bar{V}$, which has been previously investigated in animal models [70]. This approach does not require manual editing. In order to obtain a parameter that is useful in clinical practice, the second order term in Equation (7.2.1) was neglected and a linear relationship of flow velocity and pressure difference was assumed. Linear regression was applied to the data and the resulting graph was determined using the equation:

$$\Delta \bar{p} = m \cdot \bar{V} + n \qquad (7.2.2)$$

The value m denotes the slope of the linear regression, which was used as a parameter to characterize the resistance of a stenosis. The value n denotes the ordinate intercept (zero flow), which was not considered in the subsequent analysis.

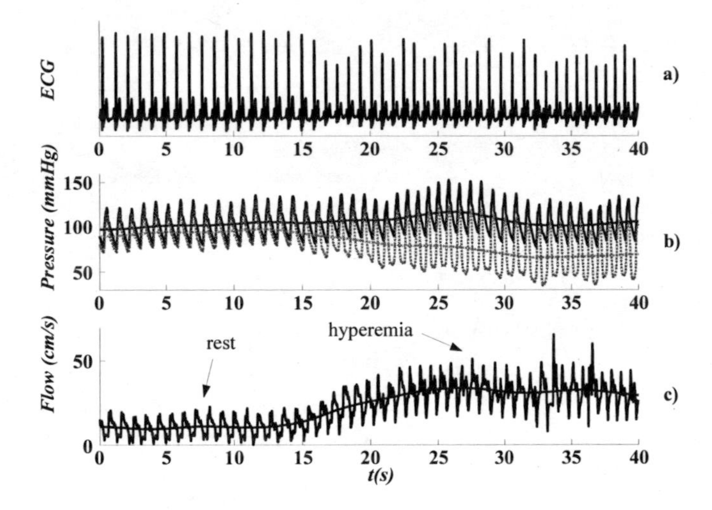

Figure 7.3: Data set consisting of (a) ECG signal, (b) proximal (solid line) and distal (dotted line) pressure signals and (c) flow velocity. The pressure and flow waveforms are plotted along with the moving average values. The arrows indicate the states of resting flow and hyperemia.

For verification purposes the results were compared to FFR, which is currently the most accurate clinically established method for functional stenosis assessment. It is defined as:

$$FFR = \frac{\bar{p}_d}{\bar{p}_a} \quad (7.2.3)$$

Here, $\bar{p}_d$ and $\bar{p}_a$ are the mean pressure values proximal and distal of a stenosis, measured at maximum hyperemia. Stenoses with $FFR < 0.75$ are considered functionally significant [7] and usually treated by percutaneous transluminal coronary angioplasty (PTCA), which involves the dilation of an artery with a balloon.

7.2.2 Spectral analysis of pressure signals

For the derivation of the parameter based on pressure measurements only, signal windows at resting conditions and at maximum hyperemia were evaluated separately. This was done in order to test the hypothesis that, in contrast to FFR, hyperemia is not a prerequisite for this method.

Spectral analysis is motivated by the fact that the pressure waveforms p_a and p_d are identical in the absence of a stenosis, while the waveforms differ in the presence of a stenosis. This is illustrated in Figure 7.4. Plot a) shows a case with a mild stenosis, the pressure waveforms are similar. In plot b) the waveforms differ in shape in the presence of a stenosis. This effect can be observed in most cases of significant stenoses and is also present at resting conditions. Thus, the evaluation of signal coherence yields information about the stenoses.

In this work, the coherence function [30] of the pressure signals is evaluated for the characterization of a stenosis. The coherence function is defined here as:

$$R_{ad}(f) = \frac{|C_{ad}(f)|^2}{C_{aa}(f) \cdot C_{dd}(f)} \quad (7.2.4)$$

In this equation, $C_{aa}(f)$ and $C_{dd}(f)$ denote the power spectra of the pressure signals p_a and p_d, respectively. $C_{ad}(f)$ represents the cross spectrum [86, 136] of both signals. The coherence function $R_{ad}(f)$ yields a value in the range of 0..1 for each frequency sample and is a measure of similarity of two signals. For the calculation of $R_{ad}(f)$ the signals were detrended, windowed with a Hanning window and transformed into the frequency domain by using the FFT. The frequency range of the signals was limited from 0..10 Hz for coherence analysis. In order to obtain a single value parameter useful for clinical practice, the mean value of the coherence function was calculated:

$$R_{mean} = \bar{R}_{ad}(f)|_{f \leq 10\,\mathrm{Hz}} \quad (7.2.5)$$

The results were again compared to the FFR values.

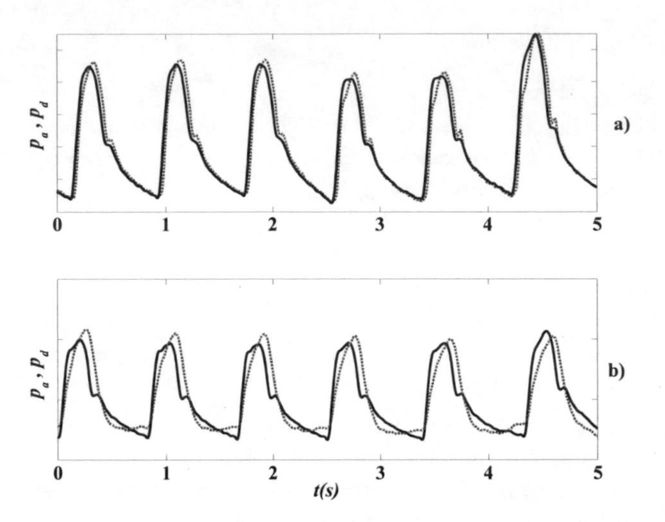

Figure 7.4 Proximal (solid lines) and distal (dotted lines) pressure waveforms at resting flow conditions. The offset of all waveforms is removed. a): Mild stenosis, the wave forms are similar. b): Hemodynamic significant stenosis, the waveforms differ in shape.

7.3 Results and discussion

The severity of the examined stenoses ranged from mild to severe obstructions, with FFR values between 0.96 and 0.55. In all patients maximum hyperemia was induced by intravenous infusion of adenosine. In Figure 7.5 the mean pressure difference is plotted versus the mean flow velocity. Six data sets are exemplarily shown. In each set the flow ranges from resting conditions to hyperemia (see Figure 7.3). The maximum flow velocity at hyperemia varies for each patient. Due to the presence of stenoses the pressure difference also rises. The graphs reflect different degrees of hemodynamic significance. Stenosis resistance changes from moderate to high with increasing slope, which was verified by FFR. The correlation of the linear regression is $r > 0.9$ for all graphs.

Figure 7.6 illustrates the correlation of the slope m with the hemodynamic significance of a stenosis. Measurements of one patient before and after PTCA are shown. Before intervention, the stenosis resistance is high. The increase in flow as a response to adenosine is minimal, but causes a significant pressure difference ($FFR = 0.55$).After angioplasty, the influence of the stenosis is reduced. The flow velocity reaches a maximum of 22 cm/s and the pressure difference is reduced ($FFR = 0.94$).

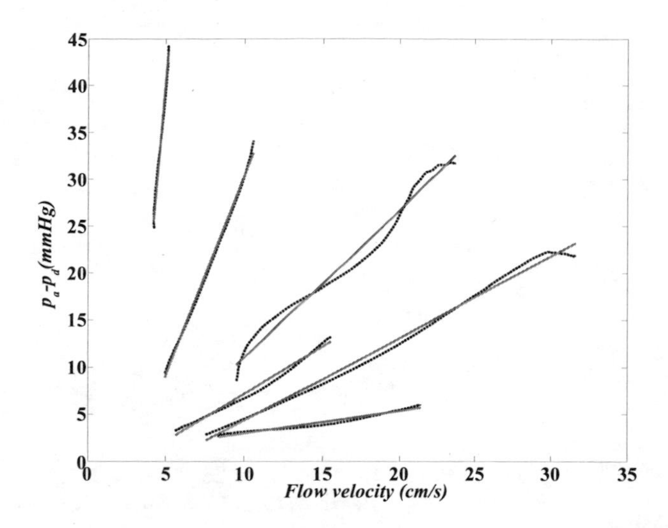

Figure 7.5: Flow-pressure gradient relationship for 6 patients with different degrees of obstruction. Linear regression (solid lines) is applied to the data (dotted lines).

Figure 7.7 shows the comparison of the estimated slopes m with FFR for all 24 measurements. The results show a correlation between FFR and the slope of the mean flow-pressure difference relationship $(r=0.65)$. As expected, the slopes increase with stenosis severity. This suggests that the flow-pressure relationship derived from mean values is a useful indicator to characterize functional stenoses severity. The evaluation of mean values is a robust method that does not require manual editing. Furthermore, the slope as a single parameter for lesion assessment seems to be sufficient and more convenient as opposed to the analysis of 2nd order polynomials.

It is known from fluid dynamics that the simultaneous measurement of pressure and flow velocity describes a lesion most accurately [71, 72]. Thus, this method has advantages in comparison to FFR in some cases, especially where hyperemia cannot be induced. This fact cannot be shown in this study, however, because FFR is currently the best validated physiological index. In order to verify the advantages of combined pressure and flow measurements, additional clinical trials with larger patient populations and a combination of different imaging modalities are needed.

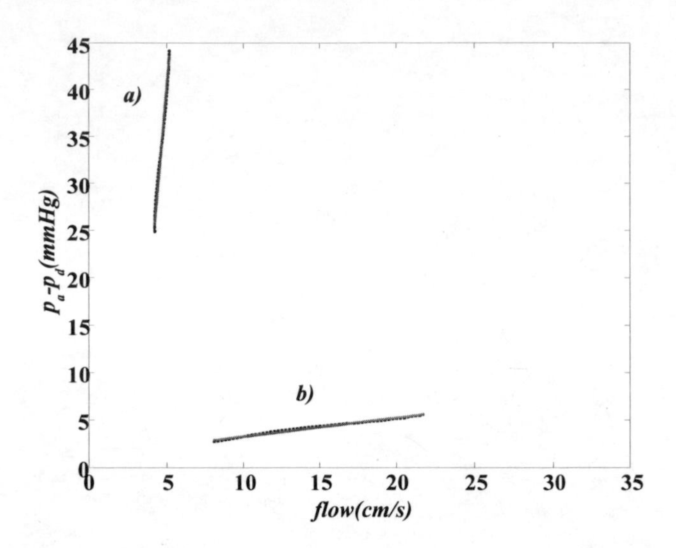

Figure 7.6: Flow-pressure gradient relationship for one patient before (a) and after balloon dilation (b). Linear regression (solid lines) is applied to the data (dotted lines).

The results for the coherence analysis are shown in Figure 7.8. Here, the mean coherence is plotted versus FFR for resting conditions and the state of maximum hyperemia. The linear regressions show a correlation of $r=0.68$ and $r=0.59$, respectively. FFR was measured at maximum hyperemia conditions in both cases, because the evaluation of FFR at resting conditions yields erroneous results [153].

The mean coherence decreases with lower FFR values as shown in both plots in Figure 7.8. The evaluation at maximum flow shows a lower correlation with the regression curve than at resting conditions. The results at resting conditions suggest that coherence analysis can provide a useful parameter also for the non-hyperemic state. Thus, it can be used in cases where maximum hyperemia cannot be induced.

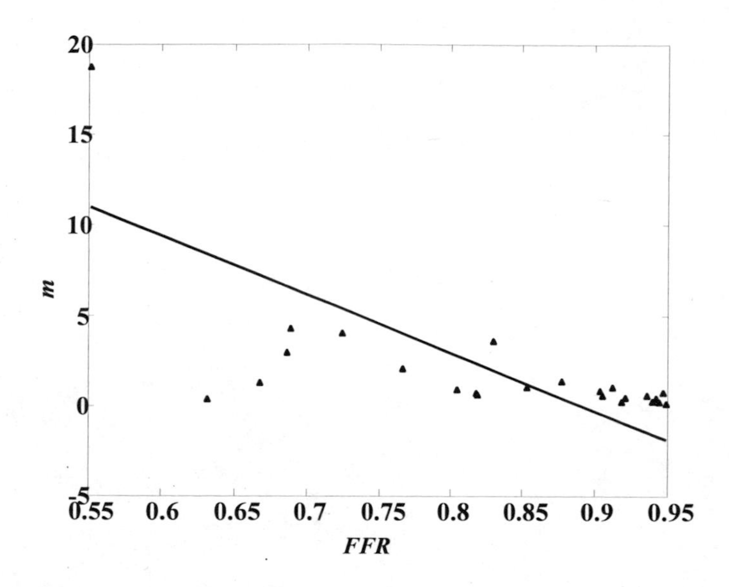

Figure 7.7: Estimated slopes m plotted versus FFR (linear regression with $r = 0.65$).

The spectral evaluation of pressure signals was previously investigated by Brosh et al. [18]. This approach evaluates high frequency components in the region of the dichrotic notch, which is characteristic for arterial pressure waveforms. However, sometimes intracoronary pressure measurements do not show a prominent dichrotic notch. In those cases the coherence analysis is more accurate because this method does not require the selection of a region within a pressure cycle.

For both developed methods, the results of this initial study show only a trend in comparison to FFR. Future work has be dedicated to the quantification of the parameters derived in this work. The final goal is a cutoff value, that characterizes stenoses as hemodynamically significant. Again, a larger patient population is needed in order to corroborate the usefulness of these methods. In comparison with the best validated approach in the evaluation of coronary artery stenosis severity (FFR), upcoming clinical trials will have to determine suitable threshold values as guidelines for clinical decisions for subsequent interventional procedures.

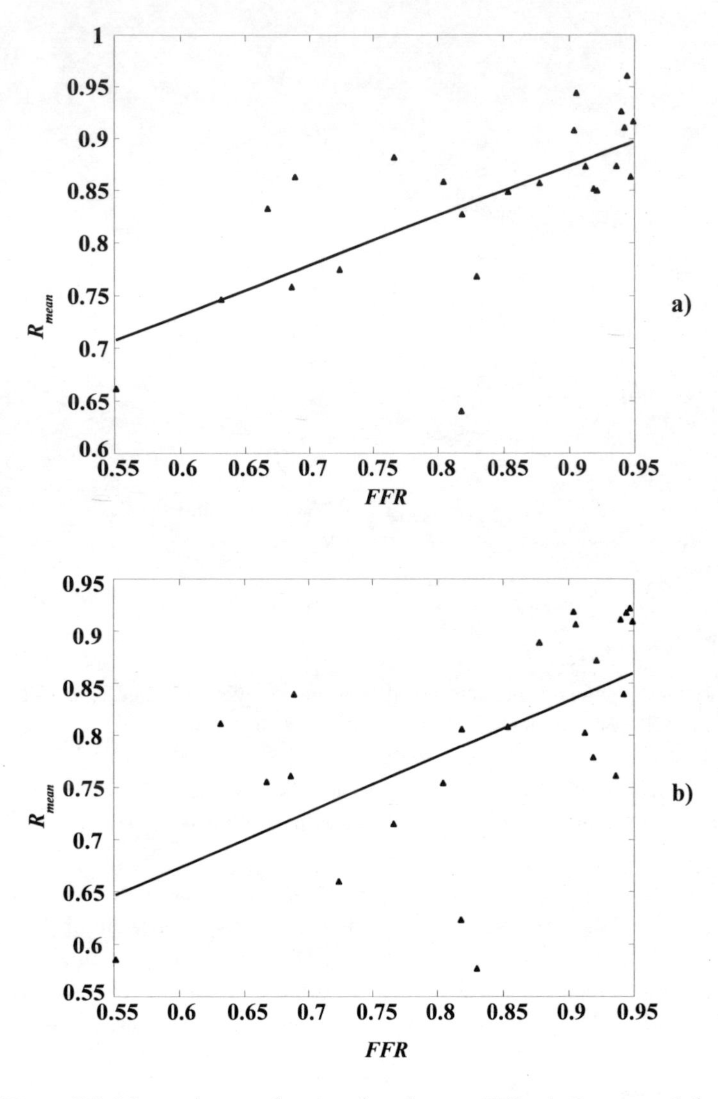

Figure 7.8: Mean coherence function plotted versus FFR. a): Data recorded at resting conditions (linear regression with $r = 0.68$). b): Data recorded at maximum hyperemia (linear regression with $r = 0.59$).

7.4 Summary

This work presented first clinical results of intracoronary pressure and blood flow velocity analysis for the assessment of coronary stenosis severity. The slope of the flow-pressure relationship calculated from mean values was used as a parameter for stenosis characterization. This evaluation method proved to be robust and did not require manual editing. The slope was shown to be correlated with FFR, which suggests that this parameter can be applied in clinical practice.

Furthermore, spectral analysis of pressure waveforms was investigated. The mean coherence function of pressure waveforms proximal and distal to a stenosis showed a correlation to FFR both at resting conditions and maximum hyperemia. Therefore, this parameter can potentially be used in cases where induction of hyperemia is not possible. This has to be verified in subsequent clinical studies with a higher patient population.

8 Summary

In this work, new methods for the assessment of coronary artery diseases with intravascular ultrasound (IVUS) were developed. The main focus of the reported methods, instrumentation and studies was on the characterization of coronary plaques with strain imaging techniques, where the mechanical properties of vessel tissue are evaluated.

After giving a short medical background and an overview of coronary imaging modalities, IVUS imaging technology was described in detail. The state of the art in catheter technology was outlined with advantages and disadvantages of single element transducers versus array technology. Intravascular Doppler measurements and instrumentation were presented briefly.

Furthermore, an introduction to IVUS strain imaging was given. the mechanical behavior of vessel walls was illustrated with a simplified cylindric model. It was shown that radial displacement as well as strain are a function of the radial distance, which has to be taken into account when interpreting strain images. The strain imaging algorithm used throughout this work was explained in detail. It estimates radial tissue displacement and strain by evaluating the phase of complex cross correlation functions using radio frequency (rf) data. The algorithm can be implemented efficiently and is real-time capable. It was also shown that the performance of this recursive algorithm depends on an initial shift value that has to be determined in order to avoid phase aliasing. For this task, accurate segmentation of the vessel walls is required as a preprocessing step.

In order to verify the performance of the algorithm with IVUS, studies were performed with circular array transducers. Ultrasound beams were formed from single channel data using synthetic aperture focusing techniques (SAFT). Phantom experiments and simulations showed that strain imaging is feasible with data reconstructed from single channel acquisitions. The main advantage of the array transducers is the absence of motion artifacts caused by mechanical rotation. However, offline beam forming was time consuming and the ultrasound signals provided by the available system showed poor SNR. Further studies should only be performed with systems that provide beamformed rf-data, which were not available during this work.

The simulations illustrated that an eccentric catheter position leads to systematic errors in the strain estimate with IVUS strain imaging. A new method for correcting these artifacts was presented using a modified synthetic aperture focusing technique, where ultrasound beams are refocused in direction of the radial strain. The results showed that this method can correct systematic strain errors due to an eccentric catheter position. The application of this approach for clinical use is limited, because in heterogeneous vessel tissue the direction of stress cannot be expected to be radial in all cases.

Furthermore, experimental studies with rotating single element transducers were performed. The main advantages of this technology are a high resolution and online accessibility of rf-data. A system for continuous acquisition of rf-data was developed that allowed the real-time calculation of strain images with up to 7 frames per second. Images acquired with rotating transducers exhibit non-uniform rotational distortion (NURD). This effect degrades the correlation of consecutive images, which poses a limitation for strain imaging. The influence of NURD was investigated experimentally in phantom studies. No significant relationship was found between catheter angulation and NURD. The degree of NURD rather depended on the mechanical properties of the individual catheters and the motor drive. In some cases the correlation of consecutive data sets was not sufficient. This fact is an important limitation for strain analysis in vivo, since the sterile equipment cannot be tested prior to the examination. It was shown in phantom experiments that decorrelation due to NURD can be reduced by beam realignment.

The performance of the strain imaging algorithms in conjunction with single element transducers was investigated in vitro and in vivo. Phantom experiments showed the feasibility of the chosen strain imaging approach under controlled conditions. Further in vitro experiments were performed with excised arteries. Calcified plaque regions were successfully identified as regions of low strain by visual comparison to the ultrasound images. Arteries with plaques identified as vulnerable were not available during this study and histologic analysis was not performed. Thus, the ability to detect these types of plaques with the proposed strain imaging approach has yet to be proven. Further in vitro studies are required to correlate strain images with histologic findings. A successful in vivo application was also demonstrated. The results suggest that 1-D radial strain estimation is feasible, but the algorithms should be enhanced. In the future, more robust algorithms for motion correction or 2-D strain estimation should be developed for further clinical trials.

Extended clinical strain imaging trials require the automated segmentation of the coronary vessel walls. In this work, two approaches for vessel wall segmentation were investigated. The first method comprised a computationally efficient segmentation method for the detection of luminal borders based on deformable models. The frame to frame decorrelation properties of flowing blood were evaluated for vessel wall detection. The normalized correlation coefficient of consecutive frames and its gradient were directly used as image forces for energy minimizing deformable models. Two algorithms were implemented and compared: A dynamic programming approach and a greedy algorithm which minimizes contour energies locally. Their performance was verified with IVUS data acquired in vivo during a clinical trial and compared to contours drawn manually by clinical experts. The results show a good agreement of manually and automatically segmented contours. The segmentation results strongly depend on the choice of contour weights, as with all deformable models. However, the computational efficiency of the implemented algorithms is a clear advantage for the use in a clinical environment.

The second presented method allowed fully automated segmentation of blood and vessel tissue based on the evaluation of spectral and textural image features. This approach was verified with data from an in vivo clinical trial. Manual segmentation was used as a gold standard. The parameters were evaluated and classified using a fuzzy inference system, which was trained and validated with 40 data sets from 4 patients. Regions containing blood or tissue were discriminated with high accuracy. The evaluation process is computationally intensive and only adequate for offline calculations. However, once the system is trained, no user interaction is required.

Finally, a concept was developed for the assessment of stable coronary plaques which form stenotic lesions. Simultaneous intracoronary pressure and blood flow velocity measurements in vivo were evaluated for the assessment of coronary stenosis severity. The slope of the flow-pressure relationship was used as a parameter to characterize stenosis resistance. This evaluation method proved to be robust and did not require manual editing. In addition, spectral analysis of pressure waveforms was investigated. The coherence function of pressure waveforms proximal and distal to a stenosis was evaluated. The results show a correlation to clinically established methods. Further clinical trials are required to determine suitable threshold values for the proposed parameters as guidelines for clinical decisions.

Bibliography

[1] A. A. Amini, T. E. Weymouth and R. C. Jain, "Using dynamic programming for solving variational problems in vision", *IEEE Transactions on Pattern Analysis and Machine Intelligence*, vol. 12, no. 9, pp. 855-867, 1990.

[2] B. A. J. Angelsen, "Ultrasound imaging", Emantec, 2000.

[3] A. Arbab-Zadeh, A. DeMaria, W. Penny, R. Russo, B. Kimura and V. Bhargava, "Axial movement of the intravascular ultrasound probe during the cardiac cycle: Implications for three-dimensional reconstruction and measurements of coronary dimensions", *Am Heart J*, vol. 138, no. 5, pp. 865-872, 1999.

[4] R. R. Archer, "An introduction to the mechanics of solids", 2 ed., McGraw-Hill, 1978.

[5] R. L. Armentano, J. Levenson, J. G. Barra, E. I. Fischer et al., "Assessment of elastin and collagen contribution to aortic elasticity in conscious dogs", *AJP - Heart and Circulatory Physiology*, vol. 260, no. 6, pp. H1870-H1877, 1991.

[6] R. L. Armentano, J. G. Barra, J. Levenson, A. Simon and R. H. Pichel, "Arterial Wall Mechanics in Conscious Dogs : Assessment of Viscous, Inertial, and Elastic Moduli to Characterize Aortic Wall Behavior", *Circulation Research*, vol. 76, no. 3, pp. 468-478, 1995.

[7] G. J. Bech, H. Droste, N. H. Pijls, B. De Bruyne et al., "Value of fractional flow reserve in making decisions about bypass surgery for equivocal left main coronary artery disease", *Heart (British Cardiac Society)*, vol. 86, no. 5, pp. 547-552, 2001.

[8] C. R. Becker, A. Knez, B. Ohnesorge, U. J. Schoepf and M. F. Reiser, "Imaging of Noncalcified Coronary Plaques Using Helical CT with Retrospective ECG Gating", *American Journal of Roentgenology*, vol. 175, no. 2, pp. 423-424, 2000.

[9] M. Bilgen, M. F. Insana, T. J. Hall and P. Chaturvedi, "Statistical analysis of strain images estimated from overlapped and filtered echo signals", *Ultrasonic Imaging*, vol. 19, no. 3, pp. 209-220, 1997.

[10] M. Bilgen and M. F. Insana, "Error analysis in acoustic elastography. II. Strain estimation and SNR analysis", *Journal of the Acoustical Society of America*, vol. 101, no. 2, pp. 1147-1154, 1997.

[11] L. N. Bohs and G. E. Trahey, "A novel method for angle independent ultrasonic imaging of blood flow and tissue motion", *IEEE Transactions on Biomedical Engineering*, vol. 38, no. 3, pp. 280-286, 1991.

[12] W. Bojara, C. Perrey, M. Lindstaedt, T. Fadgyas, B. Lemke and H. Ermert, "Charakterisierung des funktionellen Schweregrades von Koronarstenosen anhand simultaner intrakoronarer Druck- und Flussgeschwindigkeitsmessungen", *Biomedizinische Technik*, vol. 46, Suppl. 1 pp. 352-353, 2001.

[13] N. Bom, H. ten Hoff, C. T. Lancee, W. J. Gussenhoven and J. G. Bosch, "Early and recent intraluminal ultrasound devices", *International Journal of Cardiac Imaging*, vol. 4, no. 2-4, pp. 79-88, 1989.

[14] N. Bom, S. G. Carlier, A. F. W. van der Steen and C. T. Lancee, "Intravascular scanners", *Ultrasound in Medicine & Biology*, vol. 26, no. 1, pp. S6-S9, 2000.

[15] G. Braeker, "Implementierung und Verifikation eines Verfahrens zur Abbildung der mechanischen Eigenschaften von Gefäßwänden mit intravaskulärem Ultraschall", Diplomarbeit, Fakultät für Elektrotechnik und Informationstechnik, Ruhr Universität Bochum, 2001.

[16] S. L. Bridal, B. Beyssen, P. Fornes, P. Julia and G. Berger, "Multiparametric attenuation and backscatter images for characterization of carotid plaque", *Ultrasonic Imaging*, vol. 22, no. 1, pp. 20-34, 2000.

[17] I. N. Bronstein and K. A. Semendjajew, "Taschenbuch der Mathematik", 25 ed., McGraw-Hill, 1991.

[18] D. Brosh, S. T. Higano, M. J. Slepian, H. I. Miller et al., "Pulse transmission coefficient: a novel nonhyperemic parameter for assessing the physiological significance of coronary artery stenoses", *Journal of the American College of Cardiology*, vol. 39, no. 6, pp. 1012-1019, 2002.

[19] B. G. Brown, E. Bolson, M. Frimer and H. T. Dodge, "Quantitative coronary arteriography: estimation of dimensions, hemodynamic resistance, and atheroma mass of coronary artery lesions using the arteriogram and digital computation", *Circulation*, vol. 55, no. 2, pp. 329-337, 1977.

[20] B. G. Brown, X. Q. Zhao, D. E. Sacco and J. J. Albers, "Lipid lowering and plaque regression. New insights into prevention of plaque disruption and clinical events in coronary disease", *Circulation*, vol. 87, no. 6, pp. 1781-1791, 1993.

[21] E. Brusseau, C. Perrey, P. Delachartre, M. Vogt, D. Vray and H. Ermert, "Axial strain imaging using a local estimation of the scaling factor from RF ultrasound signals", *Ultrasonic Imaging*, vol. 22, no. 2, pp. 95-107, 2000.

[22] E. Brusseau, J. Fromageau, G. Finet, P. Delachartre and D. Vray, "Axial strain imaging of intravascular data: results on polyvinyl alcohol cryogel phantoms and carotid artery", *Ultrasound in Medicine & Biology*, vol. 27, no. 12, pp. 1631-1642, 2001.

[23] E. Brusseau, J. Fromageau, N. G. Rognin, P. Delachartre and D. Vray, "Investigating elastic properties of soft biological tissues", *IEEE Engineering in Medicine and Biology Magazine*, vol. 21, no. 4, pp. 86-94, 2002.

[24] C. B. Burckhardt, P. A. Grandchamp and H. Hoffmann, "An experimental 2 MHz synthetic aperture sonar system intended for medical use", *IEEE Transactions on Sonics and Ultrasonics*, vol. SU_21, no. 1, pp. 1-6, 1974.

[25] A. P. Burke, A. Farb, G. T. Malcom, Y. h. Liang, J. Smialek and R. Virmani, "Coronary Risk Factors and Plaque Morphology in Men with Coronary Disease Who Died Suddenly", *The New England Journal of Medicine*, vol. 336, no. 18, pp. 1276-1282, 1997.

[26] E. I. Cespedes, C. L. de Korte and A. F. W. van der Steen, "Echo decorrelation from displacement gradients in elasticity and velocity estimation", *IEEE Transactions on Ultrasonics Ferroelectrics & Frequency Control*, vol. 46, no. 4, pp. 791-801, 1999.

[27] E. I. Cespedes, C. L. de Korte and A. F. van der Steen, "Intraluminal ultrasonic palpation: assessment of local and cross-sectional tissue stiffness", *Ultrasound in Medicine & Biology*, vol. 26, no. 3, pp. 385-396, 2000.

[28] I. Cespedes, M. Insana and J. Ophir, "Theoretical bounds on strain estimation in elastography", *IEEE Transactions on Ultrasonics Ferroelectrics & Frequency Control*, vol. 42, no. 5, pp. 969-972, 1995.

[29] J. S. Chae, A. F. Brisken, G. Maurer and R. J. Siegel, "Geometric accuracy of intravascular ultrasound imaging", *Journal of the American Society of Echocardiography*, vol. 5, no. 6, pp. 577-587, 1992.

[30] R. E. Challis and R. I. Kitney, "Biomedical signal processing (in four parts). Part 3. The power spectrum and coherence function", *Medical & Biological Engineering & Computing*, vol. 29, no. 3, pp. 225-241, 1991.

[31] C. D. Choi, A. R. Skovoroda, S. Y. Emelianov and M. O'Donnell, "An integrated compliant balloon ultrasound catheter for intravascular strain imaging", *IEEE Transactions on Ultrasonics Ferroelectrics & Frequency Control*, vol. 49, no. 11, pp. 1552-1560, 2002.

[32] C. I. Christodoulou, C. S. Pattichis, M. Pantziaris and A. Nicolaides, "Texture-based classification of atherosclerotic carotid plaques", *IEEE Transactions on Medical Imaging*, vol. 22, no. 7, pp. 902-912, 2003.

[33] K. C. Chu and B. K. Rutt, "Polyvinyl alcohol cryogel: an ideal phantom material for MR studies of arterial flow and elasticity", *Magnetic Resonance in Medicine*, vol. 37, no. 2, pp. 314-319, 1997.

[34] B. De Bruyne, N. H. J. Pijls, L. Smith, M. Wievegg and G. R. Heyndrickx, "Coronary Thermodilution to Assess Flow Reserve: Experimental Validation", *Circulation*, vol. 104, no. 17, pp. 2003-2006, 2001.

[35] C. L. de Korte, E. I. Cespedes, A. F. van der Steen and C. T. Lancee, "Intravascular elasticity imaging using ultrasound: feasibility studies in phantoms", *Ultrasound in Medicine & Biology*, vol. 23, no. 5, pp. 735-746, 1997.

[36] C. L. de Korte, A. F. van der Steen, E. I. Cespedes and G. Pasterkamp, "Intravascular ultrasound elastography in human arteries: initial experience in vitro", *Ultrasound in Medicine & Biology*, vol. 24, no. 3, pp. 401-408, 1998.

[37] C. L. de Korte, E. I. Cespedes, A. F. van der Steen, G. Pasterkamp and N. Bom, "Intravascular ultrasound elastography: assessment and imaging of elastic properties of diseased arteries and vulnerable plaque", *European Journal of Ultrasound*, vol. 7, no. 3, pp. 219-224, 1998.

[38] C. L. de Korte, E. I. Cespedes and A. F. van der Steen, "Influence of catheter position on estimated strain in intravascular elastography", *IEEE Transactions on Ultrasonics Ferroelectrics & Frequency Control*, vol. 46, no. 3, pp. 616-625, 1999.

[39] C. L. de Korte, G. Pasterkamp, A. F. van der Steen, H. A. Woutman and N. Bom, "Characterization of plaque components with intravascular ultrasound elastography in human femoral and coronary arteries in vitro", *Circulation*, vol. 102, no. 6, pp. 617-623, 2000.

[40] C. L. de Korte and A. F. van der Steen, "Intravascular ultrasound elastography: an overview", *Ultrasonics*, vol. 40, pp. 859-865, 2002.

[41] C. L. de Korte, M. J. Sierevogel, F. Mastik, C. Strijder et al., "Identification of atherosclerotic plaque components with intravascular ultrasound elastography in vivo: a Yucatan pig study", *Circulation*, vol. 105, no. 14, pp. 1627-1630, 2002.

[42] C. L. de Korte, S. G. Carlier, F. Mastik, A. F. van der Steen, P. W. Serruys and N. Bom, "Morphological and mechanical information of coronary arteries obtained with intravascular elastography; feasibility study in vivo.", *European Heart Journal*, vol. 23, no. 5, pp. 405-413, 2002.

[43] S. A. De Winter, R. Hamers, M. Degertekin, K. Tanabe et al., "Retrospective image-based gating of intracoronary ultrasound images for improved quantitative analysis: the intelligate method", *Catheterization & Cardiovascular Interventions*, vol. 61, no. 1, pp. 84-94, 2004.

[44] P. Delachartre, C. Cachard, G. Finet, F. L. Gerfault and D. Vray, "Modeling geometric artefacts in intravascular ultrasound imaging", *Ultrasound in Medicine & Biology*, vol. 25, no. 4, pp. 567-575, 1999.

[45] J. Dijkstra, G. Koning and J. H. Reiber, "Quantitative measurements in IVUS images", *International Journal of Cardiac Imaging*, vol. 15, no. 6, pp. 513-522, 1999.

[46] Doppler, C., "Ueber das farbige Licht der Doppelsterne und einiger anderer Gestirne des Himmels," in Lorenz, H. A. (ed.), *Abhandlungen von Christian Doppler,* Verlag Wilhelm Engelmann, Leipzig, 1907.

[47] J. W. Doucette, P. D. Corl, H. M. Payne, A. E. Flynn et al., "Validation of a Doppler guide wire for intravascular measurement of coronary artery flow velocity", *Circulation*, vol. 85, no. 5, pp. 1899-1911, 1992.

[48] M. M. Doyley, F. Mastik, C. L. de Korte, S. G. Carlier et al., "Advancing intravascular ultrasonic palpation toward clinical applications", *Ultrasound in Medicine & Biology*, vol. 27, no. 11, pp. 1471-1480, 2001.

[49] M. R. Elliott and A. J. Thrush, "Measurement of resolution in intravascular ultrasound images", *Physiological Measurement*, vol. 17, no. 4, pp. 259-265, 1996.

[50] C. E. Engeler, E. R. Ritenour and K. Amplatz, "Axial and lateral resolution of rotational intravascular ultrasound: in vitro observations and diagnostic implications", *Cardiovascular & Interventional Radiology*, vol. 18, no. 4, pp. 239-242, 1995.

[51] E. Falk, P. K. Shah and V. Fuster, "Coronary Plaque Disruption", *Circulation*, vol. 92, no. 3, pp. 657-671, 1995.

[52] A. Farb, A. P. Burke, A. L. Tang, Y. Liang et al., "Coronary Plaque Erosion Without Rupture Into a Lipid Core : A Frequent Cause of Coronary Thrombosis in Sudden Coronary Death", *Circulation*, vol. 93, no. 7, pp. 1354-1363, 1996.

[53] Z. A. Fayad, V. Fuster, J. T. Fallon, T. Jayasundera et al., "Noninvasive In Vivo Human Coronary Artery Lumen and Wall Imaging Using Black-Blood Magnetic Resonance Imaging", *Circulation*, vol. 102, no. 5, pp. 506-510, 2000.

[54] Z. A. Fayad and V. Fuster, "Clinical Imaging of the High-Risk or Vulnerable Atherosclerotic Plaque", *Circulation Research*, vol. 89, no. 4, pp. 305-316, 2001.

[55] Z. A. Fayad, V. Fuster, K. Nikolaou and C. Becker, "Computed Tomography and Magnetic Resonance Imaging for Noninvasive Coronary Angiography and Plaque Imaging: Current and Potential Future Concepts", *Circulation*, vol. 106, no. 15, pp. 2026-2034, 2002.

[56] W. F. Fearon, H. M. O. Farouque, L. B. Balsam, D. T. Cooke et al., "Comparison of Coronary Thermodilution and Doppler Velocity for Assessing Coronary Flow Reserve", *Circulation*, vol. 108, no. 18, pp. 2198-2200, 2003.

[57] E. J. Feleppa, R. D. Ennis, P. B. Schiff, C. S. Wuu et al., "Spectrum-analysis and neural networks for imaging to detect and treat prostate cancer", *Ultrasonic Imaging*, vol. 23, no. 3, pp. 135-146, 2001.

[58] A. Fettweis, "Elemente nachrichtentechnischer Systeme", Teubner, 1990.

[59] G. Finet, E. Maurincomme, A. Tabib, R. J. Crowley et al., "Artifacts in intravascular ultrasound imaging: analyses and implications", *Ultrasound in Medicine & Biology*, vol. 19, no. 7, pp. 533-547, 1993.

[60] G. Finet, C. Cachard, P. Delachartre, E. Maurincomme and J. Beaune, "Artifacts in intravascular ultrasound imaging during coronary artery stent implantation", *Ultrasound in Medicine & Biology*, vol. 24, no. 6, pp. 793-802, 1998.

[61] T. Flohr, A. Kuttner, H. Bruder, K. Stierstorfer et al., "Performance evaluation of a multi-slice CT system with 16-slice detector and increased gantry rotation speed for isotropic submillimeter imaging of the heart", *Herz*, vol. 28, no. 1, pp. 7-19, 2003.

[62] G. D. Forney, "The Viterbi Algorithm", *Proceedings of the IEEE*, vol. 61, no. 3, pp. 268-278, 1973.

[63] F. S. Foster, G. R. Lockwood, L. K. Ryan, K. A. Harasiewicz, L. Berube and A. M. Rauth, "Principles and applications of ultrasound backscatter microscopy", *IEEE Transactions on Ultrasonics Ferroelectrics & Frequency Control*, vol. 40, no. 5, pp. 608-617, 1993.

[64] F. S. Foster, D. A. Knapik, J. C. Machado, L. K. Ryan and S. E. Nissen, "High-frequency intracoronary ultrasound imaging.", *Seminars in Interventional Cardiology*, vol. 2, no. 1, pp. 33-41, 1997.

[65] J. Fromageau, P. Delachartre, J. C. Boyer, R. El Guerjouma and G. Gimenez, "Modeling and measurement of cryogel elasticity properties for calibrating of IVUS elasticity images", *Proceedings of the IEEE Ultrasonics Symposium*, vol.2 pp. 1821-1824, 2000.

[66] J. Fromageau, E. Brusseau, D. Vray, G. Gimenez and P. Delachartre, "Characterization of PVA cryogel for intravascular ultrasound elasticity imaging", *IEEE Transactions on Ultrasonics Ferroelectrics & Frequency Control*, vol. 50, no. 10, pp. 1318-1324, 2003.

[67] J. G. Fujimoto, S. A. Boppart, G. J. Tearney, B. E. Bouma, C. Pitris and M. E. Brezinski, "High resolution in vivo intra-arterial imaging with optical coherence tomography", *Heart*, vol. 82, no. 2, pp. 128-133, 1999.

[68] Y. C. Fung, "Biomechanics", 2 ed., Springer-Verlag, 1993.

[69] L. Gao, K. J. Parker, R. M. Lerner and S. F. Levinson, "Imaging of the elastic properties of tissue--a review", *Ultrasound in Medicine & Biology*, vol. 22, no. 8, pp. 959-977, 1996.

[70] K. L. Gould, K. Lipscomb and C. Calvert, "Compensatory changes of the distal coronary vascular bed during progressive coronary constriction", *Circulation*, vol. 51, no. 6, pp. 1085-1094, 1975.

[71] K. L. Gould, "Pressure-flow characteristics of coronary stenoses in unsedated dogs at rest and during coronary vasodilation", *Circulation Research*, vol. 43, no. 2, pp. 242-253, 1978.

[72] K. L. Gould, "Coronary artery stenosis and reversing atherosclerosis", 2 ed., Arnold, 1999.

[73] A. Gronningsaeter, B. A. J. Angelsen, A. Gresli and H. G. Torp, "Blood noise reduction in intravascular ultrasound imaging", *IEEE Transactions on Ultrasonics Ferroelectrics & Frequency Control*, vol. 42, no. 2, pp. 200-209, 1995.

[74] A. Gronningsaeter, B. A. J. Angelsen, A. Heimdal and H. G. Torp, "Vessel wall detection and blood noise reduction in intravascular ultrasound imaging", *IEEE Transactions on Ultrasonics Ferroelectrics & Frequency Control*, vol. 43, no. 3, pp. 359-369, 1996.

[75] C. Haas, H. Ermert, S. Holt, P. Grewe, A. Machraoui and J. Barmeyer, "Segmentation of 3D intravascular ultrasonic images based on a random field model", *Ultrasound in Medicine & Biology*, vol. 26, no. 2, pp. 297-306, 2000.

[76] S. E. Hardt, A. Just, R. Bekeredjian, W. Kubler, H. R. Kirchheim and H. F. Kuecherer, "Aortic pressure-diameter relationship assessed by intravascular ultrasound: experimental validation in dogs", *AJP - Heart and Circulatory Physiology*, vol. 276, no. 3, pp. H1078-H1085, 1999.

[77] I. A. Hein and W. D. O'Brien, Jr., "Current time-domain methods for assessing tissue motion by analysis from reflected ultrasound echoes-a review", *IEEE Transactions on Ultrasonics Ferroelectrics & Frequency Control*, vol. 40, no. 2, pp. 84-102, 1993.

[78] D. Hiller and H. Ermert, "System analysis of ultrasound reflection mode computerized tomography", *IEEE Trans.Sonics, Ultrason.*, vol. SU-31, no. 4, pp. 240-250, 1984.

[79] B. K. P. Horn and B. G. Schunck, "Determining Optical-Flow", *Artificial Intelligence*, vol. 17, no. 1, pp. 185-203, 1981.

[80] A. Itoh, S. Miyazaki, H. Nonogi, S. Daikoku and K. Haze, "Angioscopic Prediction of Successful Dilatation and of Restenosis in Percutaneous Transluminal Coronary Angioplasty : Significance of Yellow Plaque", *Circulation*, vol. 91, no. 5, pp. 1389-1396, 1995.

[81] A. K. Jain, "Fundamentals of digital image processing", Prentice-Hall, London, 1989.

[82] C. R. Janssen, C. L. de Korte, M. S. van der Heiden et al., "Angle matching in intravascular elastography", *Ultrasonics*, vol. 38, no. 1-8, pp. 417-423, 2000.

[83] S. K. Jespersen, J. E. Wilhjelm and H. Sillesen, "Multi-angle compound imaging", *Ultrasonic Imaging*, vol. 20, no. 2, pp. 81-102, 1998.

[84] F. Kallel and M. Bertrand, "Tissue elasticity reconstruction using linear perturbation method", *IEEE Transactions on Medical Imaging*, vol. 15, no. 3, pp. 299-313, 1996.

[85] F. Kallel and J. Ophir, "A least-squares strain estimator for elastography", *Ultrasonic Imaging*, vol. 19, no. 3, pp. 195-208, 1997.

[86] K. D. Kammeyer and K. Kroschel, "Digitale Signalverarbeitung", 3 ed., Teubner, Stuttgart, 1996.

[87] M. Karaman, L. Pai-Chi and M. O'Donnell, "Synthetic aperture imaging for small scale systems", *IEEE Transactions on Ultrasonics Ferroelectrics & Frequency Control*, vol. 42, no. 3, pp. 429-442, 1995.

[88] M. Kass, A. Witkin and D. Terzopoulos, "Snakes: Active contour models", *International Journal of Computer Vision*, vol. 1, no. 4, pp. 321-331, 1988.

[89] P. P. Kearney, M. P. Ramo, T. Spencer, T. R. Shaw et al., "A study of the quantitative and qualitative impact of catheter shaft angulation in a mechanical intravascular ultrasound system", *Ultrasound in Medicine & Biology*, vol. 23, no. 1, pp. 87-93, 1997.

[90] M. J. Kern and B. Meier, "Evaluation of the Culprit Plaque and the Physiological Significance of Coronary Atherosclerotic Narrowings", *Circulation*, vol. 103, no. 25, pp. 3142-3149, 2001.

[91] B. J. Kimura, V. Bhargava, W. Palinski, R. J. Russo and A. N. DeMaria, "Distortion of intravascular ultrasound images because of nonuniform angular velocity of mechanical-type transducers", *American Heart Journal*, vol. 132, no. 2 Pt 1, pp. 328-336, 1996.

[92] J. D. Klingensmith, R. Shekhar and D. G. Vince, "Evaluation of three-dimensional segmentation algorithms for the identification of luminal and medial-adventitial borders in intravascular ultrasound images", *IEEE Transactions on Medical Imaging*, vol. 19, no. 10, pp. 996-1011, 2000.

[93] N. Komiyama, G. J. Berry, M. L. Kolz, A. Oshima et al., "Tissue characterization of atherosclerotic plaques by intravascular ultrasound radiofrequency signal analysis: an in vitro study of human coronary arteries.", *American Heart Journal*, vol. 140, no. 4, pp. 565-574, 2000.

[94] A. F. Kopp, S. Schroeder, A. Baumbach, A. Kuettner et al., "Non-invasive characterisation of coronary lesion morphology and composition by multislice CT: first results in comparison with intracoronary ultrasound", *European Radiology*, vol. 11, no. 9, pp. 1607-1611, 2001.

[95] G. Kovalski, R. Beyar, R. Shofti and H. Azhari, "Three-dimensional automatic quantitative analysis of intravascular ultrasound images", *Ultrasound in Medicine & Biology*, vol. 26, no. 4, pp. 527-537, 2000.

[96] E. Krestel, "Bildgebende Systeme für die medizinische Diagnostik", 2 ed., Siemens, Berlin, 1988.

[97] H. Kuttruff, "Physik und Technik des Ultraschalls", S. Hirzel Verlag, Stuttgart, 1988.

[98] K. G. Lehmann, R. J. van Suylen, J. Stibbe, C. J. Slager et al., "Composition of Human Thrombus Assessed by Quantitative Colorimetric Angioscopic Analysis", *Circulation*, vol. 96, no. 9, pp. 3030-3041, 1997.

[99] M. L. Li and P. C. Li, "Filter-based synthetic transmit and receive focusing", *Ultrasonic Imaging*, vol. 23, no. 2, pp. 73-89, 2001.

[100] W. Li, C. von Birgelen, C. Di Mario, E. Boersma et al., "Semi-automatic contour detection for volumetric quantification of intracoronary ultrasound", *Computers in Cardiology*, pp. 277-280, 1994.

[101] W. Li, A. F. van der Steen, C. T. Lancee, J. Honkoop, E. J. Gussenhoven and N. Bom, "Temporal correlation of blood scattering signals in vivo from radiofrequency intravascular ultrasound", *Ultrasound in Medicine & Biology*, vol. 22, no. 5, pp. 583-590, 1996.

[102] W. Li, A. F. van der Steen, C. T. Lancee, I. Cespedes and N. Bom, "Blood flow imaging and volume flow quantitation with intravascular ultrasound", *Ultrasound in Medicine & Biology*, vol. 24, no. 2, pp. 203-214, 1998.

[103] P. Libby, "Molecular Bases of the Acute Coronary Syndromes", *Circulation*, vol. 91, no. 11, pp. 2844-2850, 1995.

[104] M. Lindstaedt, M. K. Fritz, A. Yazar, C. Perrey et al., "Optimizing Revascularization Strategies in Patients with Multi-Vessel Coronary Disease: Impact of Intracoronary Pressure Measurements", *Journal of Thoracic and Cardiovascular Surgery*, vol. 129, no. 4, pp. 897-903, 2005.

[105] F. L. Lizzi, M. Greenebaum, E. J. Feleppa, M. Elbaum and D. J. Coleman, "Theoretical framework for spectrum analysis in ultrasonic tissue characterization", *Journal of the Acoustical Society of America*, vol. 73, no. 4, pp. 1366-1373, 1983.

[106] F. L. Lizzi, M. Ostromogilsky, E. J. Feleppa, M. C. Rorke and M. M. Yaremko, "Relationship of ultrasonic spectral parameters to features of tissue microstructure", *IEEE Transactions on Ultrasonics Ferroelectrics & Frequency Control*, vol. 34, no. 3, pp. 319-329, 1987.

[107] F. L. Lizzi, M. Astor, E. J. Feleppa, M. Shao and A. Kalisz, "Statistical framework for ultrasonic spectral parameter imaging", *Ultrasound in Medicine & Biology*, vol. 23, no. 9, pp. 1371-1382, 1997.

[108] S. Lobregt and M. A. Viergever, "A discrete dynamic contour model", *IEEE Transactions on Medical Imaging*, vol. 14, no. 1, pp. 12-24, 1995.

[109] G. R. Lockwood, L. K. Ryan, J. W. Hunt and F. S. Foster, "Measurement of the ultrasonic properties of vascular tissues and blood from 35-65 MHz", *Ultrasound in Medicine & Biology*, vol. 17, no. 7, pp. 653-666, 1991.

[110] A. Lorenz, "Zwei neue Verfahren zur Früherkennung von Prostatatumoren mit diagnostischem Ultraschall", Dissertation, Fakultät für Elektrotechnik und Informationstechnik, Ruhr-Universität Bochum, 1999.

[111] B. D. MacNeill, H. C. Lowe, M. Takano, V. Fuster and I. K. Jang, "Intravascular Modalities for Detection of Vulnerable Plaque: Current Status", *Arteriosclerosis, Thrombosis & Vascular Biology*, vol. 23, no. 8, pp. 1333-1342, 2003.

[112] J. J. Mai, F. A. Lupotti and M. F. Insana, "Vascular elasticity from regional displacement estimates", *Ultrasonic Imaging*, vol. 25, no. 3, pp. 171-192, 2003.

[113] K. M. Marques, H. J. Spruijt, C. Boer, N. Westerhof, C. A. Visser and F. C. Visser, "The diastolic flow-pressure gradient relation in coronary stenoses in humans", *Journal of the American College of Cardiology*, vol. 39, no. 10, pp. 1630-1636, 2002.

[114] A. Maseri and V. Fuster, "Is There a Vulnerable Plaque?", *Circulation*, vol. 107, no. 16, pp. 2068-2071, 2003.

[115] A. L. McLeod, R. J. Watson, T. Anderson, S. Inglis et al., "Classification of arterial plaque by spectral analysis in remodelled human atherosclerotic coronary arteries", *Ultrasound in Medicine & Biology*, vol. 30, no. 2, pp. 155-159, 2004.

[116] D. S. Meier, R. M. Cothren, D. G. Vince and J. F. Cornhill, "Automated morphometry of coronary arteries with digital image analysis of intravascular ultrasound", *American Heart Journal*, vol. 133, no. 6, pp. 681-690, 1997.

[117] M. Meuwissen, M. Siebes, J. A. Spaan and J. J. Piek, "Rationale of combined intracoronary pressure and flow velocity measurements", *Zeitschrift für Kardiologie*, vol. 91, suppl. 3, pp. 108-112, 2002.

[118] M. Meuwissen, M. Siebes, S. A. Chamuleau, B. L. Eck-Smit et al., "Hyperemic stenosis resistance index for evaluation of functional coronary lesion severity", *Circulation*, vol. 106, no. 4, pp. 441-446, 2002.

[119] A. Mojsilovic, M. Popovic, N. Amodaj, R. Babic and M. Ostojic, "Automatic segmentation of intravascular ultrasound images: a texture-based approach", *Annals of Biomedical Engineering*, vol. 25, no. 6, pp. 1059-1071, 1997.

[120] M. P. Moore, T. Spencer, D. M. Salter, P. P. Kearney et al., "Characterisation of coronary atherosclerotic morphology by spectral analysis of radiofrequency signal: in vitro intravascular ultrasound study with histological and radiological validation", *Heart*, vol. 79, no. 5, pp. 459-467, 1998.

[121] W. E. Moshage, S. Achenbach, B. Seese, K. Bachmann and M. Kirchgeorg, "Coronary artery stenoses: three-dimensional imaging with electrocardiographically triggered, contrast agent-enhanced, electron- beam CT", *Radiology*, vol. 196, no. 3, pp. 707-714, 1995.

[122] M. Naghavi, P. Libby, E. Falk, S. W. Casscells et al., "From Vulnerable Plaque to Vulnerable Patient: A Call for New Definitions and Risk Assessment Strategies: Part I", *Circulation*, vol. 108, no. 14, pp. 1664-1672, 2003.

[123] A. Nair, B. D. Kuban, N. Obuchowski and D. G. Vince, "Assessing spectral algorithms to predict atherosclerotic plaque composition with normalized and raw intravascular ultrasound data", *Ultrasound in Medicine & Biology*, vol. 27, no. 10, pp. 1319-1331, 2001.

[124] A. Nair, B. D. Kuban, E. M. Tuzcu, P. Schoenhagen, S. E. Nissen and D. G. Vince, "Coronary Plaque Classification With Intravascular Ultrasound Radiofrequency Data Analysis", *Circulation*, vol. 106, no. 17, pp. 2200-2206, 2002.

[125] T. Neumann, "Entwicklung eines Systems zur intravaskulären Ultraschall-Elastographie unter Verwendung eines rotierenden Einzelelement-Schallwandlers", Diplomarbeit, Fakultät für Elektrotechnik und Informationstechnik, Ruhr Universität Bochum, 2001.

[126] S. E. Nissen, C. L. Grines, J. C. Gurley, K. Sublett et al., "Application of a new phased-array ultrasound imaging catheter in the assessment of vascular dimensions. In vivo comparison to cineangiography", *Circulation*, vol. 81, no. 2, pp. 660-666, 1990.

[127] S. E. Nissen and P. Yock, "Intravascular Ultrasound : Novel Pathophysiological Insights and Current Clinical Applications", *Circulation*, vol. 103, no. 4, pp. 604-616, 2001.

[128] M. O'Donnell and S. D. Silverstein, "Optimum displacement for compound image generation in medical ultrasound", *IEEE Transactions on Ultrasonics Ferroelectrics & Frequency Control*, vol. 35, no. 4, pp. 470-476, 1988.

[129] M. O'Donnell, A. R. Skovorada and B. M. Shapo, "Measurement of arterial wall motion using Fourier based speckle tracking algorithms", *Proceedings of the IEEE Ultrasonics Symposium*, pp. 1101-1104, 1991.

[130] M. O'Donnell and L. J. Thomas, "Efficient synthetic aperture imaging from a circular aperture with possible application to catheter-based imaging", *IEEE Transactions on Ultrasonics Ferroelectrics & Frequency Control*, vol. 39, no. 3, pp. 366-380, 1992.

[131] M. O'Donnell, A. R. Skovoroda, B. M. Shapo and S. Y. Emelianov, "Internal displacement and strain imaging using ultrasonic speckle tracking", *IEEE Transactions on Ultrasonics Ferroelectrics & Frequency Control*, vol. 41, no. 3, pp. 314-325, 1994.

[132] M. O'Donnell, B. M. Shapo, M. J. Eberle and D. N. Stephens, "Experimental studies on an efficient catheter array imaging system", *Ultrasonic Imaging*, vol. 17, no. 2, pp. 83-94, 1995.

[133] M. O'Donnell, M. J. Eberle, D. N. Stephens, J. L. Litzza, K. San Vicente and B. M. Shapo, "Synthetic phased arrays for intraluminal imaging of coronary arteries", *IEEE Transactions on Ultrasonics Ferroelectrics & Frequency Control*, vol. 44, no. 3, pp. 714-721, 1997.

[134] B. Ohnesorge, T. Flohr, S. Schaller, K. Klingenbeck-Regn et al., "The technical bases and uses of multi-slice CT", *Radiologe*, vol. 39, no. 11, pp. 923-931, 1999.

[135] J. Ophir, I. Cespedes, H. Ponnekanti, Y. Yazdi and X. Li, "Elastography: a quantitative method for imaging the elasticity of biological tissues", *Ultrasonic Imaging*, vol. 13, no. 2, pp. 111-134, 1991.

[136] A. V. Oppenheim and R. W. Schafer, "Zeitdiskrete Signalverarbeitung", 3 ed., Oldenbourg, 1999.

[137] A. Papoulis, "Probability, random variables and stochastic processes", 3 ed., McGraw-Hill, 1991.

[138] K. J. Parker, S. R. Huang, R. A. Musulin and R. M. Lerner, "Tissue response to mechanical vibrations for "sonoelasticity imaging"", *Ultrasound in Medicine & Biology*, vol. 16, no. 3, pp. 241-246, 1990.

[139] G. Pasterkamp, E. Falk, H. Woutman and C. Borst, "Techniques characterizing the coronary atherosclerotic plaque: influence on clinical decision making?", *Journal of the American College of Cardiology*, vol. 36, no. 1, pp. 13-21, 2000.

[140] C. Perrey, "Entwicklung eines Konzeptes zur Abbildung der mechanischen Dehnung am menschlichen Rücken mit Ultraschall", Diplomarbeit, Fakultät für Elektrotechnik und Informationstechnik, Ruhr Universität Bochum, 1998.

[141] C. Perrey, G. Braeker, W. Bojara and H. Ermert, "Ein Elastographie-System zur Charakterisierung Koronarer Plaques mit Intravaskulärem Ultraschall", *Biomedizinische Technik*, vol. 46, Suppl. 1 pp. 66-67, 2001.

[142] C. Perrey, W. Wilkening, B. Brendel and H. Ermert, "A modified synthetic aperture focusing technique for the correction of geometric artefacts in intravascular ultrasound elastography", *Proceedings of the IEEE Ultrasonics Symposium*, vol. 2 pp. 1585-1588, 2001.

[143] C. Perrey, T. Neumann, W. Bojara, S. Holt and H. Ermert, "Real time intravascular ultrasound elastography with rotating single element transducers", *Proceedings of the IEEE Ultrasonics Symposium*, vol. 2, pp. 1913-1916, 2002.

[144] C. Perrey, G. Braeker, W. Bojara, M. Lindstaedt, S. Holt and H. Ermert, "Strain imaging with intravascular ultrasound array scanners: validation with phantom experiments", *Biomedizinische Technik*, vol. 48, no. 5, pp. 135-140, 2003.

[145] C. Perrey, W. Bojara, M. Lindstaedt, C. Fischer and H. Ermert, "Evaluation of intracoronary pressure and blood flow velocity for the assessment of coronary stenoses severity", *Computers in Cardiology*, pp. 247-250, 2003.

[146] C. Perrey, U. Scheipers, W. Bojara, M. Lindstaedt, S. Holt and H. Ermert, "Computerized segmentation of blood and luminal borders in intravascular ultrasound", *Proceedings of the IEEE Ultrasonics Symposium*, vol. 2 pp. 1122-1125, 2004.

[147] C. Perrey and H. Ermert, "Correction of non-uniform rotational artefacts in intravascular ultrasound elastography", *Biomedizinische Technik*, vol. 49, suppl. 2, pp. 870-871, 2004.

[148] A. Pesavento, C. Perrey, M. Krueger and H. Ermert, "A time-efficient and accurate strain estimation concept for ultrasonic elastography using iterative phase zero estimation", *IEEE Transactions on Ultrasonics Ferroelectrics & Frequency Control*, vol. 46, no. 5, pp. 1057-1067, 1999.

[149] A. Pesavento, "Quantitative Ultraschallabbildungsverfahren für die Muskeldiagnostik", Dissertation, Fakultät für Elektrotechnik und Informationstechnik, Ruhr-Universität Bochum, 1999.

[149a] A. Pesavento, A. Lorenz and H. Ermert, "System for real-time elastography", *Electronics Letters*, vol. 35, no. 11, pp. 941-942, 1999.

[150] A. Pesavento, A. Lorenz, S. Siebers and H. Ermert, "New real-time strain imaging concepts using diagnostic ultrasound", *Physics in Medicine & Biology*, vol. 45, no. 6, pp. 1423-1435, 2000.

[151] N. H. Pijls, J. A. van Son, R. L. Kirkeeide, B. De Bruyne and K. L. Gould, "Experimental basis of determining maximum coronary, myocardial, and collateral blood flow by pressure measurements for assessing functional stenosis severity before and after percutaneous transluminal coronary angioplasty", *Circulation*, vol. 87, no. 4, pp. 1354-1367, 1993.

[152] N. H. Pijls, B. De Bruyne, K. Peels, P. H. Van Der Voort et al., "Measurement of fractional flow reserve to assess the functional severity of coronary-artery stenoses.", *New England Journal of Medicine*, vol. 334, no. 26, pp. 1703-1708, 1996.

[153] N. H. Pijls and B. De Bruyne, "Coronary Pressure", 2nd ed., Kluwer Academic Publishers, 2000.

[154] N. H. Pijls, B. De Bruyne, G. J. Bech, F. Liistro et al., "Coronary pressure measurement to assess the hemodynamic significance of serial stenoses within one coronary artery: validation in humans", *Circulation*, vol. 102, no. 19, pp. 2371-2377, 2000.

[155] O. Pujol, D. Rotger, P. Radeva, O. Rodriguez and J. Mauri, "Near real-time plaque segmentation of IVUS", *Computers in Cardiology*, pp. 69-72, 2003.

[156] L. Rabiner and B. Juang, "An introduction to hidden Markov models", *IEEE ASSP Magazine*, vol. 3, no. 1, pp. 4-16, 1986.

[157] F. Rakebrandt, D. C. Crawford, D. Havard, D. Coleman and J. P. Woodcock, "Relationship between ultrasound texture classification images and histology of atherosclerotic plaque", *Ultrasound in Medicine & Biology*, vol. 26, no. 9, pp. 1393-1402, 2000.

[158] M. Rayner and S. Petersen, "European cardiovascular disease statistics", British Heart Foundation, London, 2000.

[159] K. P. Rentrop, "Thrombi in Acute Coronary Syndromes : Revisited and Revised", *Circulation*, vol. 101, no. 13, pp. 1619-1626, 2000.

[160] R. Righetti, S. Srinivasan and J. Ophir, "Lateral resolution in elastography", *Ultrasound in Medicine & Biology*, vol. 29, no. 5, pp. 695-704, 2003.

[161] J. Ed. Roelandt, "Intravascular Ultrasound", Kluwer Academic Publishers, 1993.

[162] L. K. Ryan, G. R. Lockwood, B. G. Starkoski, D. W. Holdsworth et al., "A high frequency intravascular ultrasound imaging system for investigation of vessel wall properties", *Proceedings of the IEEE Ultrasonics Symposium*, pp. 1101-1105, 1992.

[163] L. K. Ryan, G. R. Lockwood, T. S. Bloomfield and F. S. Foster, " Speckle tracking in high frequency ultrasound images with application to intravascular imaging", *Proceedings of the IEEE Ultrasonics Symposium*, pp. 889-892, 1993.

[164] L. K. Ryan and F. S. Foster, "Ultrasonic measurement of differential displacement and strain in a vascular model", *Ultrasonic Imaging*, vol. 19, no. 1, pp. 19-38, 1997.

[165] Y. Saijo and A. F. van der Steen, "Vascular Ultrasound", Springer Verlag, 2003.

[166] J. A. Schaar, C. L. de Korte, F. Mastik, R. Baldewsing et al., "Intravascular palpography for high-risk vulnerable plaque assessment", *Herz*, vol. 28, no. 6, pp. 488-495, 2003.

[167] J. A. Schaar, C. L. de Korte, F. Mastik, C. Strijder et al., "Characterizing vulnerable plaque features with intravascular elastography", *Circulation*, vol. 108, no. 21, pp. 2636-2641, 2003.

[168] U. Scheipers, H. Ermert, H. J. Sommerfeld, M. Garcia-Schurmann, T. Senge and S. Philippou, "Ultrasonic multifeature tissue characterization for prostate diagnostics", *Ultrasound in Medicine & Biology*, vol. 29, no. 8, pp. 1137-1149, 2003.

[169] U. Scheipers, H. Ermert, H. J. Sommerfeld, M. Garcia-Schurmann et al., "Ultrasonic tissue characterization for prostate diagnostics: spectral parameters vs. texture parameters", *Biomedizinische Technik*, vol. 48, no. 5, pp. 122-129, 2003.

[170] U. Scheipers, "Methods and system for ultrasonic tissue characterization based on a multifeature approach and fuzzy inference systems", Dissertation, Fakultät für Elektrotechnik und Informationstechnik, Ruhr Universität Bochum, 2004.

[171] W. Schmidt, M. Niendorf, D. Maschke, D. Behrend, K. P. Schmitz and W. Urbaszek, "Analysis of intravascular ultrasound (IVUS) echo signals for characterization of vessel wall properties", *Acoustical Imaging*, vol. 24, pp. 295-300, 2000.

[172] G. Schmitz, H. Ermert and T. Senge, "Tissue-characterization of the prostate using radio frequency ultrasonic signals", *IEEE Transactions on Ultrasonics Ferroelectrics & Frequency Control*, vol. 46, no. 1, pp. 126-138, 1999.

[173] K. Schröder, "Implementierung und Optimierung der rekonstruktiven intravaskulären Ultraschallabbildung mit synthetischer Apertur", Diplomarbeit, Fakultät für Elektrotechnik und Informationstechnik, Ruhr Universität Bochum, 1998.

[174] B. M. Shapo, J. R. Crowe, A. R. Skovoroda, M. J. Eberle, N. A. Cohn and M. O'Donnell, "Displacement and strain imaging of coronary arteries with intraluminal ultrasound", *IEEE Transactions on Ultrasonics Ferroelectrics & Frequency Control*, vol. 43, no. 2, pp. 234-246, 1996.

[175] B. M. Shapo, J. R. Crowe, R. Erkamp, S. Y. Emelianov, M. J. Eberle and M. O'Donnell, " Strain imaging of coronary arteries with intraluminal ultrasound: experiments on an inhomogeneous phantom", *Ultrasonic Imaging*, vol. 18, no. 3, pp. 173-191, 1996.

[176] M. Siebes, B. J. Verhoeff, M. Meuwissen, R. J. de Winter, J. A. Spaan and J. J. Piek, "Single-wire pressure and flow velocity measurement to quantify coronary stenosis hemodynamics and effects of percutaneous interventions", *Circulation*, vol. 109, no. 6, pp. 756-762, 2004.

[177] A. R. Skovoroda, S. Y. Emelianov and M. O'Donnell, "Tissue elasticity reconstruction based on ultrasonic displacement and strain images", *IEEE Transactions on Ultrasonics Ferroelectrics & Frequency Control*, vol. 42, no. 4, pp. 747-765, 1995.

[178] M. Sonka, Z. Xiangmin, M. Siebes, M. S. Bissing et al., "Segmentation of intravascular ultrasound images: a knowledge-based approach", *IEEE Transactions on Medical Imaging*, vol. 14, no. 4, pp. 719-732, 1995.

[179] M. Sonka, V. Hlavac, and R. Boyle, "Image processing, analysis and machine vision", 2nd ed., Brooks/Cole, 1998.

[180] T. Spencer, M. P. Ramo, D. M. Salter, T. Anderson et al., "Characterisation of atherosclerotic plaque by spectral analysis of intravascular ultrasound: an in vitro methodology", *Ultrasound in Medicine & Biology*, vol. 23, no. 2, pp. 191-203, 1997.

[181] S. Srinivasan, R. Righetti and J. Ophir, "Trade-offs between the axial resolution and the signal-to-noise ratio in elastography", *Ultrasound in Medicine & Biology*, vol. 29, no. 6, pp. 847-866, 2003.

[182] Statistisches Bundesamt Deutschland. Sterbefälle nach den 10 häufigsten Todesursachen. http://www.destatis.de , 2004.

[183] C. Stefanadis, L. Diamantopoulos, C. Vlachopoulos, E. Tsiamis et al., "Thermal heterogeneity within human atherosclerotic coronary arteries detected in vivo: A new method of detection by application of a special thermography catheter", *Circulation*, vol. 99, no. 15, pp. 1965-1971, 1999.

[184] C. Stefanadis, K. Toutouzas, E. Tsiamis, C. Pitsavos, L. Papadimitriou and P. Toutouzas, "Identification and stabilization of vulnerable atherosclerotic plaques: the role of coronary thermography and external heat delivery", *Indian Heart Journal*, vol. 53, no. 1, pp. 104-109, 2001.

[185] C. Stefanadis, K. Toutouzas, M. Vavuranakis, E. Tsiamis, S. Vaina and P. Toutouzas, "New balloon-thermography catheter for in vivo temperature measurements in human coronary atherosclerotic plaques: a novel approach for thermography?", *Catheterization & Cardiovascular Interventions*, vol. 58, no. 3, pp. 344-350, 2003.

[186] M. Sugeno and T. Yasukawa, "A fuzzy-logic-based approach to qualitative modeling", *IEEE Transactions on Fuzzy Systems*, vol. 1, no. 1, pp. 7, 1993.

[187] C. Sumi, A. Suzuki and K. Nakayama, "Estimation of shear modulus distribution in soft tissue from strain distribution", *IEEE Transactions on Biomedical Engineering*, vol. 42, no. 2, pp. 193-202, 1995.

[188] A. Takagi, K. Hibi, X. Zhang, T. J. Teo et al., "Automated contour detection for high-frequency intravascular ultrasound imaging: a technique with blood noise reduction for edge enhancement", *Ultrasound in Medicine & Biology*, vol. 26, no. 6, pp. 1033-1041, 2000.0

[189] H. E. Talhami, L. S. Wilson and M. L. Neale, "Spectral tissue strain: a new technique for imaging tissue strain using intravascular ultrasound", *Ultrasound in Medicine & Biology*, vol. 20, no. 8, pp. 759-772, 1994.

[190] G. J. Tearney, M. E. Brezinski, B. E. Bouma, S. A. Boppart et al., "In Vivo Endoscopic Optical Biopsy with Optical Coherence Tomography", *Science*, vol. 276, no. 5321, pp. 2037-2039, 1997.

[191] H. Ten Hoff, A. Korbijn, T. H. Smith, J. F. Klinkhamer and N. Bom, "Imaging artifacts in mechanically driven ultrasound catheters", *International Journal of Cardiac Imaging*, vol. 4, pp. 195-199, 1989.

[192] S. P. Timoshenko and J. N. Goodier, "Theory of Elasticity", McGraw-Hill, 1970.

[193] J. M. Tobis, J. Mallery, D. Mahon, K. Lehmann et al., "Intravascular ultrasound imaging of human coronary arteries in vivo. Analysis of tissue characterizations with comparison to in vitro histological specimens", *Circulation*, vol. 83, no. 3, pp. 913-926, 1991.

[194] E. J. Topol and S. E. Nissen, "Our Preoccupation With Coronary Luminology : The Dissociation Between Clinical and Angiographic Findings in Ischemic Heart Disease", *Circulation*, vol. 92, no. 8, pp. 2333-2342, 1995.

[195] P. A. Tunick, G. A. Krinsky, V. S. Lee and I. Kronzon, "Diagnostic Imaging of Thoracic Aortic Atherosclerosis", *American Journal of Roentgenology*, vol. 174, no. 4, pp. 1119-1125, 2000.

[196] M. S. van der Heiden, M. G. de Kroon, N. Bom and C. Borst, "Ultrasound backscatter at 30 MHz from human blood: influence of rouleau size affected by blood modification and shear rate", *Ultrasound in Medicine & Biology*, vol. 21, no. 6, pp. 817-826, 1995.

[197] A. F. van der Steen, J. M. Thijssen, J. A. van der Laak, G. P. Ebben and P. C. de Wilde, "Correlation of histology and acoustic parameters of liver tissue on a microscopic scale", *Ultrasound in Medicine & Biology*, vol. 20, no. 2, pp. 177-186, 1994.

[198] R. J. M. van Geuns, P. A. Wielopolski, H. G. de Bruin, B. J. W. M. Rensing et al., "MR Coronary Angiography with Breath-hold Targeted Volumes: Preliminary Clinical Results", *Radiology*, vol. 217, no. 1, pp. 270-277, 2000.

[199] T. Varghese, J. Ophir and I. Cespedes, "Noise reduction in elastograms using temporal stretching with multicompression averaging", *Ultrasound in Medicine & Biology*, vol. 22, no. 8, pp. 1043-1052, 1996.

[200] T. Varghese, J. Ophir, E. Konofagou, F. Kallel and R. Righetti, "Tradeoffs in elastographic imaging", *Ultrasonic Imaging*, vol. 23, no. 4, pp. 216-248, 2001.

[201] R. Virmani, F. D. Kolodgie, A. P. Burke, A. Farb and S. M. Schwartz, "Lessons From Sudden Coronary Death : A Comprehensive Morphological Classification Scheme for Atherosclerotic Lesions", *Arteriosclerosis, Thrombosis, and Vascular Biology*, vol. 20, no. 5, pp. 1262-1275, 2000.

[202] R. Virmani, A. P. Burke, F. D. Kolodgie and A. Farb, "Vulnerable plaque: the pathology of unstable coronary lesions.", *Journal of Interventional Cardiology*, vol. 15, no. 6, pp. 439-446, 2002.

[203] M. Vogt, "Konzepte für die hochauflösende Blutflußabbildung mit hochfrequentem Ultraschall", Dissertation, Fakultät für Elektrotechnik und Informationstechnik, Ruhr Universität Bochum, 2004.

[204] D. Vray, C. Haas, T. Rastello, M. Krueger et al., "Synthetic aperture-based beam compression for intravascular ultrasound imaging", *IEEE Transactions on Ultrasonics Ferroelectrics & Frequency Control*, vol. 48, no. 1, pp. 189-201, 2001.

[205] R. F. Wagner, S. W. Smith, J. M. Sandrik and H. Lopez, "Statistics of speckle in ultrasound B-scans", *IEEE Transactions on Sonics and Ultrasonics*, vol. 30, no. 3, pp. 156-163, 1983.

[206] Waller, B., "Coronary anatomy and pathology: What the angiogram does not reveal," in Tobis, J. M. and Yock, P. G. (eds.), *Intravascular ultrasound imaging,* Churchill Livingstone, New York, 1992, pp. 17-34.

[207] M. Wan, Y. Li, J. Li, Y. Cui and X. Zhou, "Strain imaging and elasticity reconstruction of arteries based on intravascular ultrasound video images", *IEEE Transactions on Biomedical Engineering*, vol. 48, no. 1, pp. 116-120, 2001.

[208] R. J. Watson, C. C. McLean, M. P. Moore, Spencer et al., "Classification of arterial plaque by spectral analysis of in vitro radio frequency intravascular ultrasound data", *Ultrasound in Medicine & Biology*, vol. 26, no. 1, pp. 73-80, 2000.

[209] J. Weinberger, L. Ramos, J. A. Ambrose and V. Fuster, "Morphologic and dynamic changes of atherosclerotic plaque at the carotid artery bifurcation: sequential imaging by real time B-mode ultrasonography", *Journal of the American College of Cardiology*, vol. 12, no. 6, pp. 1515-1521, 1988.

[210] J. Weinberger, S. Azhar, F. Danisi, R. Hayes and M. Goldman, "A New Noninvasive Technique for Imaging Atherosclerotic Plaque in the Aortic Arch of Stroke Patients by Transcutaneous Real-Time B-Mode Ultrasonography : An Initial Report", *Stroke*, vol. 29, no. 3, pp. 673-676, 1998.

[211] W. Wilkening, "Konzepte zur Signalverarbeitung für die kontrastmittelspezifische Ultraschallabbildung", Fakultät für Elektrotechnik und Informationstechnik, Ruhr Universität Bochum, 2004.

[212] D. J. Williams and M. Shah, "A fast algorithm for active contours and curvature estimation", *CVGIP: Image Understanding*, vol. 55, no. 1, pp. 14-26, 1992.

[213] L. S. Wilson, M. L. Neale, H. E. Talhami and M. Appleberg, "Preliminary results from attenuation-slope mapping of plaque using intravascular ultrasound", *Ultrasound in Medicine & Biology*, vol. 20, no. 6, pp. 529-542, 1994.

[214] H. Yabushita, B. E. Bouma, S. L. Houser, H. T. Aretz et al., "Characterization of Human Atherosclerosis by Optical Coherence Tomography", *Circulation*, vol. 106, no. 13, pp. 1640-1645, 2002.

[215] Y. Yamakoshi, J. Sato and T. Sato, "Ultrasonic imaging of internal vibration of soft tissue under forced vibration", *IEEE Transactions on Ultrasonics Ferroelectrics & Frequency Control*, vol. 37, no. 2, pp. 45-53, 1990.

[216] J. T. Ylitalo and H. Ermert, "Ultrasound synthetic aperture imaging: monostatic approach", *IEEE Transactions on Ultrasonics Ferroelectrics & Frequency Control*, vol. 41, no. 3, pp. 333-339, 1994.

[217] X. Zhang, C. R. McKay and M. Sonka, "Tissue characterization in intravascular ultrasound images", *IEEE Transactions on Medical Imaging*, vol. 17, no. 6, pp. 889-899, 1998.

[218] Y. Zhou, G. S. Kassab and S. Molloi, "In vivo validation of the design rules of the coronary arteries and their application in the assessment of diffuse disease", *Physics in Medicine and Biology*, vol. 6, pp. 977-993, 2002.

Acknowledgments

Die vorliegende Arbeit entstand während meiner Tätigkeit als wissenschaftlicher Mitarbeiter am Lehrstuhl für Hochfrequenztechnik der Ruhr-Universität Bochum. Ich möchte all denjenigen herzlich danken, die zum erfolgreichen Abschluss dieser Arbeit beigetragen haben.

Besonders möchte ich mich bei Herrn Professor Dr.-Ing. Helmut Ermert bedanken, der meinen beruflichen Werdegang in nicht unerheblichem Maße beeinflusst hat. Von der Bearbeitung meiner Diplomarbeit über meinen Forschungsaufenthalt bei Siemens Medical Systems bis zur Realisierung des vorliegenden Textes hat Herr Professor Ermert meine Arbeiten mit großem Interesse verfolgt und unterstützt. Mit der Möglichkeit der Teilnahme an zahlreichen internationalen Konferenzen sowie der Einrichtung des Kompetenzzentrums Medizintechnik Ruhr hat er meinen Kollegen und mir ein Arbeitsumfeld mit hervorragenden Voraussetzungen für unsere Forschungsaktivitäten geschaffen.

Weiterhin danke ich Herrn Professor Dr.-Ing. Werner von Seelen herzlich für die Übernahme des Korreferats.

Den Kolleginnen und Kollegen sowie den technischen Mitarbeitern am Lehrstuhl für Hochfrequenztechnik danke ich für die gute Zusammenarbeit, die intensiven fachlichen Diskussionen und nicht zuletzt auch für die sehr freundschaftliche Atmosphäre im Team. Meinen Kollegen Michael Vogt, Mohammad Ashfaq und Bernhard Brendel danke ich für die Durchsicht des Manuskripts und die konstruktiven Hinweise zu dieser Arbeit. Meinem Kollegen Ulrich Scheipers möchte ich für die motivierenden Gespräche bei unseren gemeinsamen Konferenzteilnahmen danken.

Bedanken möchte ich mich weiterhin bei den studentischen Hilfskräften und Studienarbeitern sowie den Diplomanden Thorsten Neumann und Gudrun Braeker, die dieses Projekt mit Kreativität und hohem Arbeitseinsatz unterstützt haben.

Die beschriebenen klinischen Erprobungen fanden in enger Zusammenarbeit mit den Projektpartnern aus den Berufsgenossenschaftlichen Kliniken Bergmannsheil Bochum statt. Mein besonderer Dank gilt den beteiligten Ärzten Dr. Waldemar Bojara, Dr. Michael Lindstaedt, und Dr. Stephan Holt sowie allen Mitarbeitern der Abteilung für Kardiologie und Angiologie. Sie haben diese Arbeit mit großem Engagement begleitet und mit der Aufnahme und Bearbeitung klinischer Daten, fachlichem Rat und hoher Diskussionsbereitschaft wesentlich zu ihrer Realisierung beigetragen.